Welcome to

THE
EVERYTHING®
PARENT'S GUIDES

As a parent, you're swamped with conflicting advice and parenting techniques that tell you what is best for your child. THE EVERYTHING® PARENT'S GUIDES get right to the point about specific issues. They give you the most recent, up-to-date information on parenting trends, behavior issues, and health concerns—providing you with a detailed resource to help you ease your parenting anxieties.

THE EVERYTHING® PARENT'S GUIDES are an extension of the bestselling Everything® series in the parenting category. These family-friendly books are designed to be a one-stop guide for parents. If you want authoritative information on specific topics not fully covered in other books, THE EVERYTHING® PARENT'S GUIDES are the perfect resource to ensure that you raise a healthy, confident child.

Visit the entire Everything® series at *www.everything.com*.

THE EVERYTHING

PARENT'S GUIDE TO

Children with Juvenile Diabetes

Dear Reader,

When my youngest daughter, Lauren, was diagnosed with diabetes at her sixth birthday nearly a decade ago, I felt more alone than I ever imagined I would in my life. Diabetes was a stranger to me, and despite the 700 children in Lauren's elementary school, I had no other parent to relate to. I dug for books and searched for information and learned all I could about helping her with this new life.

After a year, I reached out and began to volunteer with the Juvenile Diabetes Research Foundation raising funds for a cure, helping with advocacy in Washington, and serving as a volunteer support person to newly diagnosed families. As the years went by, I found that while giving support, I still needed to get it too. Diabetes is ever-evolving and needs our constant attention.

I was—and am—thankful to have a world of support around me now. It is my hope that this book works like a long, comfortable conversation, or like a support group in print. Read it and let it help you. But don't stop there. Follow the theme I push from chapter to chapter: Reach out and get real-time support; reach out and make a difference. We diabetes parents need each other. Until the cure, I stand ready to help, as you all eventually will as well.

Sincerely,

Moira McCarthy

THE

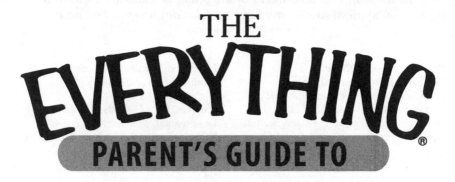

EVERYTHING®

PARENT'S GUIDE TO

CHILDREN WITH
JUVENILE
DIABETES

Reassuring advice for managing symptoms
and raising a healthy, happy child

Moira McCarthy
Technical Review by Jake Kushner, M.D.

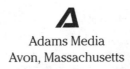

Adams Media
Avon, Massachusetts

*To the staff and volunteers of the Juvenile Diabetes Research
Foundation. And to my Lauren, who deserves to be cured.*

• • •

Publisher: Gary M. Krebs
Managing Editor: Laura M. Daly
Associate Copy Chief: Sheila Zwiebel
Acquisitions Editor: Kerry Smith
Development Editor: Brett Palana-Shanahan
Associate Production Editor: Casey Ebert

Director of Manufacturing: Susan Beale
Production Project Manager:
Michelle Roy Kelly
Prepress: Erick DaCosta, Matt LeBlanc
Design and Layout: Heather Barrett,
Brewster Brownville, Colleen Cunningham,
Jennifer Oliveira

• • •

An Everything® Series Book.
Everything® and everything.com® are registered trademarks of F+W Publications, Inc.

Published by Adams Media, an F+W Publications Company
57 Littlefield Street, Avon, MA 02322 U.S.A.
www.adamsmedia.com

ISBN 10: 1-59869-246-1
ISBN 13: 978-1-59869-246-4

Printed in Canada.

J I H G F E D C B A

Library of Congress Cataloging-in-Publication Data
McCarthy, Moira.
The everything parent's guide to children with juvenile diabetes /
Moira McCarthy, with Jake Kushner.
p. cm.—(An everything series book)
Includes index.
ISBN-13: 978-1-59869-246-4 (pbk.)
ISBN-10: 1-59869-246-1 (pbk.)
1. Diabetes in children. 2. Diabetes in children. 3. Patients—Home care. I. Kush-
ner, Jake. II. Title. III. Title: Parent's guide to children with juvenile diabetes.

RJ420.D5M385 2007
618.92'462—dc22
2007001122

*All the examples and dialogues used in this book are fictional, and have
been created by the author to illustrate medical situations.*

▶**di•a•be•tes** (díə-bē´ tĭs,-tēz) n. *also called diabetes mellitus*; **1.** a chronic condition in which the body is unable to produce insulin and properly break down sugar (glucose) in the blood, requiring the administration of insulin by external means.

Acknowledgments

How can you begin to thank a group of friends and supporters who stretch out over what seems like a lifetime of dealing with diabetes? First, all my amazing friends—both staff and volunteer—at the JDRF, especially the Public Affairs Department, the Government Relations Department, and the New England Chapter. In particular, Heidi Daniels, Kara Coen, Peter Cleary, Michele Ariano, Susan Sobers, Larry, Ronnie and Laura, Mike, Jaime and Abbie, Peter Van Etten, Cynthia Ford, Nancy Jones, Rik Bonness and family, Kassy "Marsha" Helme, Katie Clark and her curly little Mini-me, my volunteer idol Ardy, the all-knowing Mollie, the tireless Dr. S. Robert Levine, Gail Pressberg, and so many more. My online goddesses Ellen and Renee, who understand everything and are always there for me. My tennis and tanning pals at the Eel River Beach Club; my fellow members of the Spoiled Upper Middle Class Women Who Have Time to Play Tennis in the Middle of the Week League at the Kingsbury Club and across the state; the creators of Tab Energy; the staff of Children's Hospital in Boston (Dr. Jake Kushner, Susan Crowell, and Dr. Joe Wolfsdorf, the most). Good friends who listen like the Tripps, Jean Driscoll, the Husbands, and Paul and Jen; Jean and Leo Hartnett who know how to pour a drink when needed, and the many members of Lauren's League for a Cure. To my agent Gina Panettieri, who talked me into this, and to Kerry Smith of Adams Media for being a true partner. Most of all, I thank my family: husband Sean for letting me be me, Leigh for being the best daughter and big sister on earth, and Lauren, who has been a champion not just for herself, but for all who suffer with diabetes. Together, we have survived this, and together, we will beat it.

Contents

Introduction

No doubt you've found your way to this book as the parent or primary caregiver of a child who has been newly diagnosed with diabetes. It's been a worrisome time: You've had to learn all about a new and complicated disease that the world in general thinks is no big deal. You've had to begin to accept that your child's life has changed in many ways, and that your family life has been changed at its core.

But you've also realized that it's up to you, as the adult, to make this work. Your goal is to make your child's life as normal as possible while keeping him or her as healthy as possible. You know this will be a challenge, and you realize you need real-time help and support, more than just your medical team can offer.

This book is intended to be a foundation for just that. Written from one parent to another, it is a real-time, nothing-held-back, honest, and basic approach to helping you, your child, and your entire family not just cope with diabetes but thrive, because truly, there is no "magic bullet" to make your child's life easier. It's ironic: The world in general (and admit it, before your child's diagnosis, most of you thought this, too) thinks diabetes is a treatable disease, one that, with a few tweaks in lifestyle choices, pretty much fades into the background of life. Parents of children with diabetes know that is far from reality. They know that they face a lifetime of questions

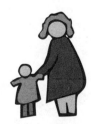

and challenges, of even day-to-day changes in their child's treatment and plan.

This book does not give you every little detail of daily care, but rather it provides an overview of what to expect in every part of your child's life with diabetes. You won't find algorithms for insulin doses, but you will find discussions on which insulin works best in different situations. You won't find a breakdown of the internal workings of each insulin pump available, but you will find information on pumping and when it is or isn't the best choice for a child.

Your reaching for this book proves that you are ready to think carefully through each aspect of your child's life with diabetes. Consider this book your friend, a place where you can ponder and reflect on the challenges you are facing, and think through new situations. This book is a support group on paper, a friend to talk things through with that is bound and printed. Keep it handy and check back on issues as they arise. Most of all use it to push yourself to a new level, where you are helping not just your own child but all families coping with diabetes. Until the cure is found, the truth is we all need each other.

CHAPTER 1

What Is Type 1 Diabetes?

For many families dealing with their child's diabetes diagnosis, even the concept of the disease and what it means is completely new. A vast majority of children have Type 1, or autoimmune, diabetes. Understanding its basics will help parents or caregivers begin to work and live with it.

The Physiology of Type 1 Diabetes

Understanding the mechanics of what causes Type 1 diabetes helps a person understand the basics of the disease, its effects, and even how it differs from other similar diseases.

How It Begins

Although no one is sure exactly what triggers the body to develop Type 1 diabetes, science and research have come a long way in getting closer to that point. Some aspects of the disease are understood, while others are still being studied.

Research has shown that the body of a person who develops Type 1 diabetes "turns against itself." The T cells of the immune system become confused and attack the body instead of protecting it. For reasons still not completely understood, the T cells attack the pancreas's beta cells, located within the Islets of Langerhans. These beta cells produce insulin to help convert food into fuel.

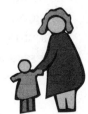

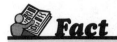 **Fact**

Until 1997, this type of diabetes was called juvenile diabetes, since it almost always affects children. But with the discovery that this disease also affects adults in rare cases, its name was changed to Type 1 diabetes.

Scientists are still trying to figure out the exact cause for the T cells' confusion. Current speculation is that a combination of a genetic irregularity and some sort of environmental trigger must be present; however, a person can have that genetic irregularity and never develop Type 1 diabetes.

The onset can be as slow as a few years or as quick as a few months. Oftentimes, parents report their child had another type of trauma—the flu, another sickness, or even an injury—at the time of onset. Although certain sicknesses or injuries can occur just before a diagnosis of Type 1 diabetes, they are not the cause of the illness. Rather, the strain of those events may have helped stimulate the onset of diabetes.

Even though it is always beneficial to catch a disease early, it is not yet possible to stop the onset of diabetes. (See Chapter 21 for details on research toward that goal.)

The Autoimmunity

As the body develops the autoimmunity, and the T cells attack and damage or destroy the islet cells, the body slowly begins to lose its ability to process food into fuel. That's because the insulin produced by these cells is the link between the body's fuel (glucose from food) and the cells. Insulin tells the body to use glucose for fuel. Without insulin, the body doesn't receive the clues that it's time to process food into fuel.

As the insulin-producing cells (the beta cells) within the Islets of Langerhans begin to die, the pancreas does not make enough insulin to store glucose properly. The person's blood sugar rises, and she begins to urinate more often as the glucose forces her body to produce more urine. The increased loss of urine causes dehydration, which she senses as increased thirst. As diabetes progresses, the insulin shortage becomes more severe, and the body goes into starvation mode. This starvation mode causes the body to break down fat for energy, which causes a by-product called ketones to build up. At this point, a scary metabolic crisis can occur, termed diabetic ketoacidosis or DKA. (See Chapter 5 for a detailed explanation of ketones.)

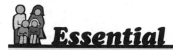 **Essential**

A great book to illustrate this autoimmunity to children and adults is *It's Time to Learn about Diabetes*, a workbook written by Jean Betschart-Roemer and published by John Wiley & Sons. This book's simple analogies help explain the process in terms that are easy for anyone to grasp.

Signs and Symptoms

After the autoimmunity begins and the islet cells slowly begin to die, the child (or person) affected begins to show signs and symptoms that can add up to a diagnosis of Type 1 diabetes. Many parents don't know the symptoms, but some lucky ones do. The sooner you can recognize the symptoms, the sooner your child can get treatment.

Obvious Signs

After a diagnosis, more than one parent has beaten themselves up about the "obvious" signs that they just didn't see. The fact is that events, trauma, and illness happen to children. Most parents are not aware of all the symptoms of Type 1 diabetes, and so they attribute the symptoms they notice as being caused by other events.

The first sign most parents or caregivers become aware of is a higher frequency of urination. Parents of small children report noticing soaked-through diapers on what seems to be a constant basis and extremely heavy diapers at changing time.

Older children will visit the restroom more often. One reason many children seem to be diagnosed on family vacations is that is a time when parents notice a child's bathroom visits. At home, a child can slip off to the powder room; on a vacation, however, Mom or Dad has to hunt down a restroom each time.

Oftentimes, a child (even a teenager) begins to experience bed-wetting. If a child has just transitioned into kindergarten or become an older sibling for the first time, parents often attribute this symptom to regression or relate it to stress.

 Essential

At the start of a diagnosis, it is important to tell a child that his or her bedwetting was a symptom of the onset of diabetes. Wetting the bed can be a source of shame or guilt for some children, so reassure your child that this bedwetting was beyond his control.

The second obvious sign is weight loss. The body cannot use food for fuel, and so it must find the fuel elsewhere. Most patients lose weight because their bodies are forced to eat away at fat and muscle for fuel. A child can drop a good amount of weight quickly, and in fact, most patients lose weight prior to diagnosis. But here again, it's easy for parents to misinterpret this symptom, thinking the weight loss is due to losing baby fat, engaging in more exercise, or just growing into a different type of body. Also, most parents don't weigh their children regularly.

Less Obvious Signs

There can be other hints that diabetes is present. Behavior changes often accompany constant high blood sugar. Many parents report "losing control" of their children just before diagnosis; the child becomes irritable, uncooperative, even sullen. These changes, on their own, would never lead a parent to think about diabetes, but combined with other symptoms, they can provide another piece of the puzzle.

Children can also develop excessive thirst or hunger before diagnosis. The thirst comes from the increased production and loss of urine, or osmotic diuresis, discussed earlier. Some children, even tiny ones, can hurriedly guzzle giant glasses of water or other drinks. Hunger comes from the body's inability to find fuel, since it is not being told to do so by the insulin. Again, parents can attribute the thirst to playing outside on a hot day and the increased appetites to a growth spurt. But the pieces of the puzzle are now beginning to fall into place.

If these signs remain undetected, more drastic symptoms such as vomiting, stomach pain, and rapid breathing can follow. These symptoms should be treated as an emergency, and immediate, hands-on care should be sought.

Type 1 Versus Type 2

Most patients with diabetes—about 90 percent of them—have Type 2. This means that most people's knowledge of diabetes is based on what they know about Type 2. Understanding the differences between the two types is crucial for parents and for anyone interacting with your child.

Autoimmune Versus Metabolic

As you will see in Chapter 2, Type 2 diabetes is a metabolic disease, not an autoimmune disease like Type 1. What this means, in simple English, is that a person with Type 1 diabetes does not produce his own insulin and never will, no matter what he does. A person with Type 2 diabetes still produces insulin, but her body has a hard time using the insulin properly and sometimes does not produce enough. This is why, with diet and exercise, a person with Type 2 diabetes can improve somewhat, while a person with Type 1 cannot.

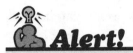

Alert!

Be ready for people who think your child has the same diabetes as their great aunt. They'll tell you that she did just fine once she cut out jelly doughnuts, and that there are pills available now to treat it. You'll need to explain the differences calmly, and you may have to accept that they won't believe you.

Another important point is that there is nothing you or your child did wrong to cause Type 1 diabetes. It does not matter how or what you eat or don't eat, or how often you exercise or don't exercise: Nothing that you control can start or stop the progression of diabetes. You will have to drive this point home to your child and to everyone who knows her. You and your child are not to blame. Similarly, although lifestyle has a powerful influence, genetic and environmental factors also are strong contributors to the risk of Type 2 diabetes.

Is It Genetic?

Everyone will ask if diabetes runs in your family. First, there is no known connection between Type 2 diabetes and Type 1 diabetes running together in a family. Most people know that Type 2 diabetes is highly familial, or genetic, so many will assume that your child's Type 1 diabetes is as well. The answer, while somewhat simple, is as complicated as everything else in this disease. Families that have a member with Type 1 diabetes do have a higher chance of another family member having Type 1, but the chance is still so low that it is not expected. In fact, only single-digit percentages of families have more than one person with Type 1 diabetes.

Type 2, on the other hand, can be quite common in family members, particularly in older adults. If you have a family member with Type 2, your physician will watch you through the years and will most likely counsel you to exercise and keep your weight down to offset the probability of Type 2 in your future.

Statistics and Type 1

The numbers are changing and growing when it comes to incidences of Type 1 diabetes, but some facts remain the same. It is, for the most part, a disease that strikes in childhood and at all ages of childhood.

Age Breakdowns

Researchers used to be able to say with all confidence that a vast majority of children with Type 1 diabetes are diagnosed around puberty. For a time, scientists believed hormonal changes might be one of the triggers for onset. Today, however, more and more children are being diagnosed at every age from two weeks to adulthood.

Although more and more infants are being diagnosed, it is still thought that only about one percent of children with diabetes are one year old or less. Fewer than 10 percent are five years old or younger.

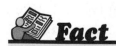 **Fact**

Statistics show that about 5 percent of the 16 million Americans with diabetes have Type 1. This percentage imbalance demonstrates why most people know about and understand only the more common Type 2 diabetes.

While practitioners are diagnosing more young children, the fact still remains that adolescents are diagnosed most often. According to Children's Hospital in Boston, which has a pediatric endocrine department, the average age of diagnosis is right around puberty—about ten to twelve years old for girls and twelve to fourteen years old for boys.

That does not mean that if your child has passed puberty, there is no chance for him to be diagnosed with diabetes. Older people, from young adults to those in their forties, are now showing signs of Type 1 diabetes. This can be shocking to an adult, and even to her medical team, because most people assume that diabetes symptoms in an adult must be Type 2. As a result, Type 2 is no longer called adult onset diabetes.

How Many Families Are Out There?

Parents often feel completely alone when their child is diagnosed with diabetes. But the fact is there are thousands of families out there just like you. While they may not be right on your street, they are certainly in your community or nearby.

One of the reasons diabetes totals can differ from source to source is that unlike other diseases, diabetes has not yet been officially tracked by the Centers for Disease Control. However, that effort is now under way as the five-year Tracking Diabetes in Youth Program, and diabetes advocates hope to have real numbers in the near future. One thing is known for sure: The numbers are growing. Pediatric diabetes centers across the nation report increases in newly diagnosed children.

If this is true, why do you and your child feel alone? With estimates of one in every 600 or so children developing Type 1 diabetes, there's a good chance your child could be the only one in his school with Type 1. But if you look farther, you'll find others.

Common Misperceptions and Truths

Few diseases have more myths and misperceptions than diabetes. Some of these misconceptions are due to the confusion between the two types of diabetes; some are due to the many recent (and still relatively unknown) advances in treating the disease. You'll need to get the facts straight for yourself first and for everyone else next.

Diabetes Can Be Regulated

After your child is diagnosed, you'll be asked more than a few times, "Is her diabetes regulated yet?" A prevalent misconception is that diabetes is a controllable disease and that, once you've figured out insulin doses and cut back on sweets, it really is not such a big deal. Parents walk a fine line between explaining the realities to the world and not frightening their children.

The truth is there is no such thing as "regulation" or "remission" in Type 1 diabetes. Because the body can never again produce its own insulin, and because injecting insulin is a rough art at best, children with Type 1 diabetes are watched vigilantly. This fact is also why the slogan of the Juvenile Diabetes Research Foundation is "insulin is not a cure."

Insulin is a great treatment, and it keeps children alive, but it does not cure diabetes. The only cure for diabetes is to find a way to induce the body to create its own insulin again.

No More Sweets!

Just about all the world will cluck in disapproval if your child eats cake or ice cream or any other treat. This is because, in the old days, it was thought people with diabetes needed to eat less sugar. But the realization in recent years that all carbohydrates break down into glucose in the body means that "a carb is a carb is a carb." In today's Type 1 care, as long as you count the carbohydrates and match them with insulin, just about any food is acceptable.

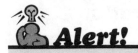
Alert!

As with any child, you'll want to teach your child to eat healthfully and limit sweets. Work with your nutritionist to figure out how often to fit sweets into the day, and when to say no. But ask him or her to make your child's eating habits as normal as possible.

This is a hard myth to crack, since so many people had elderly relatives who had to stay away from sugar. Just tell people that your child's diet is discussed with her medical team, and that new insulin and other treatments allow children to have more freedom when it comes to eating.

People will also have to understand that sometimes, a sugary food is the best thing a child with diabetes can have. Insulin doses are hard to estimate, and children can go low, and the quickest way to bring blood sugars back up from low is a sugary food. Frosting, sugary drinks, or candy are often a must.

Others will say, "As long as it's not processed sugar, it's okay," or "Natural sugar like fruit is fine." This is not true. You will need to account for every single carbohydrate your child eats.

You Could Have Avoided Diabetes

Yes, someone will say it: If only you'd fed your child right, you wouldn't be dealing with this. It's simply not true. Be strong and say it, so your child knows that you know it: Nothing you or your child did caused this autoimmune disease, and there's nothing you could have done to stop it. The only thing you can do now is learn all you can about daily care and work toward a cure.

You also need to let your child know (and you need to accept it as well) that no family history could force Type 1 to occur or avoid its onset. Some people like to say that getting diabetes is like being hit by lightning. It happens, but it's that rare and unusual.

Treatment Options

Type 1 diabetes has only one basic treatment option: replacement insulin therapy. In the past there was a strict regimented way for administering that therapy. As the years go by, however, more and more ways to do that are open to families coping with diabetes.

The Old Way

Not so long ago, children with diabetes were given one or two shots of insulin a day and strict meal plans. Today, while some children's treatments start out this way, in time and with education, every child—with the help of his or her parent or caregiver—can find a more reasonable and normal way to live with diabetes.

If your child has been on a peaking, long-acting insulin like NPH combined with a shorter-acting insulin that forces a strict adherence to eating or not eating at a certain time of day, talk to your medical team about more flexible options. (See Chapter 6 for detailed insulin choices.)

Some medical teams believe it's good to start out with the old way of doing things because it gives parents a buffer in which to learn more about diabetes until they are ready for more complicated (yet freeing) treatments. As long as your team knows you want to learn and work toward that day, they should keep you moving toward it.

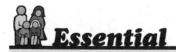

Essential

If you think your child is ready for something like an insulin pump and your medical team will not work with you, you may want to consider finding a new team. To be successful in your child's treatments, you'll need a team that is willing to match your style of care.

The old way also means a set meal plan, and this is something children love to move past quickly. It wasn't so long ago that children had to eat an exact, almost prescribed, amount of food at the same time each day. Today, that strict diet has changed.

The New Way

Now, with fast-acting insulin, nonpeaking insulin, and pumps and continuous meters, families can work toward a level of care that allows more freedom, even if it does come with more responsibility. Your best bet to move toward this goal is to let your medical team know, from the start, that you want to work with them to get your family educated and ready for the best, most humane care possible for your child. Let them know you'll be reading a lot and attending a reputable support program. Ask them to work with you toward your goal. In the end, finding the most modern, normal daily routine possible will help your child get through the years of constant care with less stress and more happiness—and that's not a small feat.

CHAPTER 2

Type 2 Diabetes and Children

U ntil recently, Type 2 diabetes, formerly known as adult onset diabetes, was thought to affect only adults, usually over forty years old. But in recent years, studies have found that in some cases, children can suffer from Type 2 diabetes as well. A look at how and why this can happen is helpful not only to those who are dealing with Type 2 but also to those children dealing with Type 1, since the differences between the two need to be understood.

The Physiology of Type 2 Diabetes

Like Type 1 diabetes, Type 2 begins with a genetic precursor. In almost all cases, there is a family history. But unlike Type 1, the environmental triggers of Type 2 diabetes are not only clear but possibly avoidable in children as well as in some adults.

When Insulin Doesn't Work

In Type 2 diabetes, the body still produces insulin, but the body's cells have trouble using it properly. Researchers are still studying why this occurs. Do the cells have a hard time recognizing the insulin? Do the cells need more insulin than a normal body for special reasons? Whatever the case, as Type 2 develops, the body begins to be unable to make the connection with the insulin available. The pancreas struggles, putting out more and more insulin. Eventually, the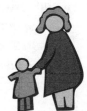

pancreas reaches a limit of how much insulin it can produce while the body still is unable to recognize the insulin available.

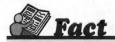 **Fact**

The term *insulin resistance* refers to the early stages of Type 2 diabetes, when the body is making plenty of insulin, but the cells are unable to use that insulin productively.

While children experiencing the onset of Type 1 diabetes often have rapid weight loss, children experiencing the onset of Type 2 diabetes usually have a weight problem, even obesity. Although when a child is experiencing constant high blood sugar from Type 2, he can lose weight as well, but it would follow a period of obesity.

How Can It Happen in Children?

Although Type 2 was thought to occur only in older bodies, some doctors are reporting more occurrences in children, particularly obese and sedentary children. While the media has made this an issue, according to the Centers for Disease Control, "a statistically significant increase in the prevalence of Type 2 diabetes among children and adolescents was found only for American Indians."

There are other claims of an increase in Latino and African-American communities as well. Studies are looking at both the genetic and lifestyle issues in these ethnic groups.

In any case, more and more pediatricians are now on the lookout for Type 2 diabetes in children. Markers include a family history, a child whose body mass index is over the 85th percentile, or a child who is over the 120th percentile in weight for her age. Children who fall into these categories are now being watched carefully and being counseled about how to avoid the disease.

Why Type 2 Is Hard for a Kid

In the world of diabetes, Type 2 sufferers are the vast majority. But in the world of kids and diabetes, Type 1 is the most prominent. The child with Type 2 finds himself dealing with a new disease, and he probably knows few peers who are in a similar situation. This can be troubling and challenging for the child and the caregiver alike.

Their Own Minority

While some studies show the number of children with Type 2 is increasing, they are still in the minority when it comes to the total number of kids with diabetes. A child with Type 2 will almost certainly not have any peers in school who have the same illness and she will have to face different challenges than a child with Type 1.

Children with Type 2 face a different challenge than those with Type 1: While children with Type 1 must change their lives to accommodate shots and blood checks, children with Type 2 usually need to make lifestyle changes, such as restrictions on their diet and a need for increased exercise. These kinds of lifestyle changes can be hard for a child, particularly if a parent is not pushing for it to happen.

That means that although kids with Type 1 can eat the same as most kids, kids with Type 2 may have to change their diet drastically. Although this can be alienating and even embarrassing for children, it must be done because noncompliance can be particularly troubling. People with Type 2, for the most part, do not go into the metabolic crisis known as diabetic ketoacidosis (DKA); they can linger at a high A1c, which is the average of their blood sugar levels over an extended period, and blood glucose average for a long time, long enough to cause complications (see Chapter 5 for more on DKA and A1c). People with Type 1 need complete insulin replacement, so they tend to slip into a dangerous place quickly and must immediately deal with their situation. Such immediacy does not apply to Type 2 sufferers; Type 2 diabetes can be damaging in the patient's ability to ignore it.

The Blame Game

As hard as it is to deflect the questions of blame when dealing with Type 1 diabetes, it's even harder with Type 2. Since so much of the reason for the disease is tied to lifestyle, weight, and activity levels, a child and her parent can feel as if they had some control in the onset of diabetes. With Type 2, blame can come along with shame; shame from parents or caregivers that they let their child's lifestyle affect her health; shame from a child for being overweight and for having a medical issue that is usually connected with the elderly.

Parents should avoid lashing out at a child who develops Type 2. The best action is to connect with a pediatric endocrinology team that specializes in Type 2 diabetes and in children and weight issues in children and then move forward, realizing that there are good solutions available.

Taking Control of Type 2

The good news is that people dealing with Type 2 diabetes, despite their genetic predisposition, are in a position to improve their situation somewhat. Step by step, Type 2 can be controlled.

Diet First

You'll want your child immediately under the care of a pediatric endocrinology team that includes a top-notch dietitian. It's not easy being a kid and changing diets, but a good dietitian can help guide a child to a lifetime of healthful eating. Oftentimes, it's a good idea to include the entire family because chances are, if a child has become obese, he's from a family that eats in relatively the same way.

A good dietitian will help your child—and your family—adapt slowly and surely to new ways of eating. Quitting cold turkey seldom works for anyone. Rather, a step-by-step plan that includes new cooking ideas, meal planning, and creative snacking is the best option.

Try to work some exciting specials into your child's new meal plan, and ask your dietitian to help you be creative. Remember, some foods that look safe may not be so; for example, sugar-free candy has carbs, too. Rather than sugar-free candies, find good, healthful snack choices that you may never have considered before.

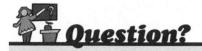 **Question?**

Are purchased diet plans a good choice for my child?
Just as you would discuss any medical decisions with your child's doctor, discuss any diet choices with your child's dietitian. Plans like Weight Watchers can be great, but some others might not be the best choice for a child.

Exercise Comes Next

As easy as it is to blame the increase of Type 2 in kids on video games, there's way more to it than that, and in fact, video games don't need to be banned completely from your child's life. If you haven't introduced sports or active playtime, now is the time to begin. But as always, take it slowly and with professional help.

If you can afford it, you may want to consider a trainer for your child. Going to the gym or even outside with a trainer may be exciting and fun for your child, and the trainer will know how slowly and safely to take your child from inactive to athlete.

If a trainer is not within your budget, ask your pediatric endocrinology team to help you outline an exercise program. It should include walking, swimming (if possible), and eventually, a new sport or two.

As for the video games, make clear limits about the amount of time they are to be played. Also you can attach other goals to the video games. For instance, if your child walks or plays actively for more than an hour and a half, he can play a video game for a half hour. Just make sure you keep the games under your control (i.e., keep them in a place where your child only has access to them through you).

You may also want to consider limiting Internet access. More than a few children now spend hours online, sitting and not getting exercise. By turning off the Internet or restricting it except for special times, you'll keep the temptation away from her.

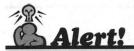

Alert!

Don't throw a child who was inactive for a lifetime immediately on to a soccer team. This can be traumatic for both the child and her body. Remember, it takes time to tone a body for sports, and you'll want to let your child adapt emotionally and physically to this new active lifestyle.

Statistics

Accurate data on the number of children with Type 2 diabetes is hard to find, but it will be easier to access in the future because the disease is being studied so closely. In the meantime, some early statistics and concepts are being published and becoming available to you.

How Many Kids Have Type 2?

No one wants to answer that yet. The study most frequently cited in the claims of massive increases in the number of kids with Type 2 is from a pharmaceutical company that ships Type 2 medications to patients. According to a study done by Express Scripts, a pharmacy benefits company, the number of children on medications for Type 1 rose 31 percent from 2002 to 2005, but the number of children on medication for Type 2 rose 104 percent during the same period. That statistic can be deceptive, since a vast majority of children are on medications for Type 1 rather than Type 2 (even though 104 percent of a small number sounds alarming, it may be statistically small compared to the Type 1 number). Still, it does show an increase and needs to be considered.

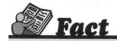**Fact**

> The Express Scripts study also reports that many children on Type 2 medications are taking them not because they currently have Type 2, but because they are deemed to be at risk for developing Type 2 in the near future.

As is the case with Type 1 diabetes, the Centers for Disease Control is attempting to assess the total number of children with diabetes. The CDC study should provide some real numbers in the near future.

Long-Term Statistics

The worrisome news is that, while they may have more of a chance to turn things around through diet and exercise, children with Type 2 seem to suffer complications at a high rate. This is partially because, like children with Type 1, their bodies are being subjected to the effects of high blood sugars from a younger age.

Also with Type 2 diabetes, some physicians suggest blood checks only twice a day; this allows blood sugars to remain elevated longer if they are up and thus permits damage to the body to occur sooner. Talk to your child's medical team about setting tougher standards of care for your child than most adults with Type 2 have. Ask for an A1c check every four months, just as a child with Type 1 would have. Remember that an A1c check is a long-term look at your child's blood sugar levels, so as long as your child's A1c is above normal (see Chapter 5 for more details on A1c levels), expect your child to check his blood sugar at least four times a day. It may be tempting to go easy on your child, but vigilance will pay off.

Treatment Options

We've talked about diet and exercise, but sometimes even more needs to be done for a child dealing with Type 2. With the help of your medical team, you can consider other options such as new medications and holistic options.

Medications

Type 2 medications are modernizing even more quickly than are medications for Type 1. The good news is that the market is huge, and pharmaceutical companies are extremely motivated to find Type 2 medications that work. Talk to your medical team. If a medication is available to help your child's insulin work better, is it a good idea? They'll consider your child's age, how long she should be on such medication, and if the plan is to work toward her not needing it anymore.

 Essential

Do not ever accept a simple medication as a solution to your child's Type 2 diabetes. Every good Type 2 plan includes a diet and fitness complement. Refuse to settle for less, and move on to another medical team if your team centers only on medication.

Some over-the-counter medications claim to help the body use glucose better. Never add any of these medications to your child's routine without getting consent from your medical team. Even Type 2 medications can sometimes cause lows, and often interaction with other medications—even over-the-counter meds—can spell trouble. As good as something may sound, always run it by your child's medical team first.

Holistic Answers

There's a push out there to "cure" diabetes with holistic solutions from acupuncture to herbs. Although it's good to look into every option, it is crucial that you never try any of these treatments without the consent and input of your child's medical team.

That's not to say there are not good holistic options. But even in the case of good options, you need to be absolutely sure that what you are considering is in the best interests of your child. In other words, never let anyone outside of your child's health team convince you to try a treatment that you don't truly know will help, not hurt, your child.

A Cure for Type 2?

It's safe to say that there is a reasonable answer to the Type 2 diabetes problem. In most cases, healthful living and eating can help bring it under control. In many cases, children with Type 2 do go on medications, and battling to live without them is not easy. But will there be a cure for Type 2? Research is being conducted to offset and even avoid the complications that make Type 2 dangerous. With good care and scientific breakthroughs, complications such as heart disease, blindness, and kidney failure—once staples of a future with Type 2 diabetes—may someday be a thing of the past. (See Chapter 21 for more discussion on breakthroughs in forestalling and treating complications.)

Support for Type 2

Unlike Type 1 diabetes, support for kids with Type 2 is harder to find. You'll need to be creative in how and where to find your support and your child's support.

Groups

Most Type 2 support groups are filled with adults and senior citizens, people your child simply will not mesh with. Most support groups for children with diabetes focus on Type 1. You and your child might not be comfortable with these groups either, since the issues are so different. Your first option is to consider a support group for kids dealing with almost the same issues as your child: obesity and lifestyle changes. It might be that your child will find support with kids trying to make the same lifestyle changes, even if they are not facing Type 2 diabetes yet.

Essential

> Consider a health camp for your child this coming summer. Don't think of it as fat camp. Think of it as a place where your child will be surrounded by kids facing the same issues as he is, and where he'll learn to better his life.

You can also ask your medical team if they hold any kind of support meetings for kids and families dealing with Type 2 diabetes. They certainly should be sensitive enough not to put you and your child into an uncomfortable situation. If such a group does not exist, perhaps it would be empowering to form one. Consider starting a group that not only sits and talks but also gets up and walks or runs or exercises, thus embracing the very activities that are necessary for healthful living with Type 2.

Online

Like anything else today, there is online support for Type 2 children and families. Childrenwithdiabetes.com has a forum for kids and parents that can be logged on to at any time, day or night. The American Diabetes Association has information on their Web site at *www.diabetes.org* about kids and diabetes. One great thing about the World Wide Web is that even though kids with Type 2 are spread around the world, they can easily find themselves in one "room," giving support and advice, and most of all, letting each other know they are not alone. As is always the case with children and the Web, monitor your child's use of the Internet and make sure the Web site he is using is well run and respected. Don't let him chat anywhere or with anyone you have not checked out first.

CHAPTER 3

Diagnosis Day

C hances are if you're reading this book, you've already experienced your child's diagnosis day. It is a day (or a series of days) that will impact you both for a long time, and what does and does not happen on that day will be replayed in your mind again and again. Your story—your "dx day," as parents of kids with diabetes call it—will become your lifetime icebreaker with other parents of kids with diabetes. Looking back on the experience and figuring out how to learn from it helps every parent or caregiver cope.

How It Happens

For a vast majority of parents, their child's diagnosis comes as a complete shock. Since the majority of people who deal with diabetes are often adults dealing with Type 2, most people's frame of reference is not a little child or a teen who suddenly becomes thin and ill. Some parents are astute enough (or have experience) to recognize the symptoms early; for them, diagnosis day may be a bit less frightening but just as upsetting. How your day goes will depend on how you came to recognize the disease.

Early Diagnosis

For parents who recognized the symptoms (many are medical professionals or have close relatives with diabetes), diagnosis day can occur before a medical crisis ever happens. Parents who know the symptoms—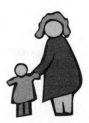

excessive thirst, frequent urination, and rapid weight loss—often receive the first real sign with the results of a home blood glucose test or a quick call to the pediatrician. Some children have even been diagnosed with blood sugars still in the high 100s, and the lower the blood sugar at diagnosis, the less stressful the immediate impact.

There are many benefits of an early diagnosis. First, your child's blood sugar will be brought down quite easily with a dose of insulin at the doctor's office. Second, early diagnosis often means a longer honeymoon period (see Chapter 14 for details). Your child may not have lost an excessive amount of weight, meaning he won't have to work at gaining it back. You may also avoid the trauma of doctors working to bring your child out of diabetic ketoacidosis (see Chapter 5 for details), a condition that, left untreated, can lead to a coma and even death.

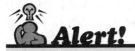

Trust your instincts. If you call your pediatrician's office and they tell you not to worry and to wait a day or so to see what comes along, insist on being seen. If they refuse, head to your local emergency room. When you're looking at a diagnosis of diabetes, it is always better to be safe than sorry.

Parents who recognize symptoms sometimes have family members or friends who have a child with diabetes. In this case, your most important tool, a support system, may be in place from the start. Let this family member or friend talk you through the whole diagnosis experience. Such help is priceless.

Later Diagnosis

For a vast majority of families, the diagnosis comes once the disease is further along. With children, diabetes is not something parents regularly consider. Although many diabetes groups are doing their best to educate the public about the symptoms of diabetes and how to recognize them, it simply is not common knowledge.

For some parents, the first hint comes from a school nurse, a teacher, or a coach. They may notice your child taking excessive bathroom breaks or going to the water fountain constantly. In the case of teachers or coaches, this may come as a criticism rather than an alert to possible trouble. Remember, they probably have as little knowledge of diabetes symptoms as you had. Be thankful that they let you know what was going on, no matter what their tone was.

Parents of toddlers and babies begin to notice that their children constantly have heavy, wet diapers and quickly drink their bottles and juice boxes. Parents of older children notice bedwetting, weight loss, and even behavior changes.

Yet, for many parents, all these signs can be written off to other causes. Parents of young children can think it is the stress of starting school. Some think that bedwetting is simply a retention issue. The behavior problems that can come from the irritability a child feels with high blood sugar are often assumed to be displays of attitude. Parents have even punished their children for these displays, not realizing that it was really a symptom of a disease.

 Essential

You must let go of any guilt you carry for not noticing your child's symptoms earlier. Remember, you could not have stopped the diabetes from coming on, and it is quite common not to recognize the symptoms. Forgive yourself and focus your energy on moving ahead.

Many diagnoses happen at annual checkups (thus the high incidence of children being diagnosed on or around their birthdays). Your pediatrician should check blood sugar and dip urine for ketones annually. Some parents, even those with no background in children and diabetes, report that as soon as the pediatrician's office tells them of their suspicions, all the pieces of the puzzle come together. It's a tough moment when you realize that your child has been critically ill right under your nose. More than one parent has not been able to hold it together at that time. If you got very upset, even in front of your child, forgive yourself and explain to your child that you were frightened for a moment and cried out, just as he or she sometimes does.

Where to Go and What to Expect

In most cases, a child's diagnosis day leads you to an inpatient experience at a city hospital with a pediatric endocrinology department. In some cases, families are actually sent home with insulin and directed to an outpatient training program that begins the next day. In some very rare cases, families are given a few hours of training and then sent home with the telephone number of a doctor to call for help. Which will you be? Some of it is actually in your control. If you did not have the type of diagnosis experience that sent you home ready to deal with this, it's never too late to consider starting again.

The Pediatrician

The first place most parents turn (and rightfully so) is their primary care pediatrician. This is the person you have the most comfortable relationship with; and in many cases, this is the person who must refer you to a specialist for insurance reasons. Your pediatrician has the tools to diagnose your child. He or she can do a blood sugar check and ketone urine dip right in the office and let you know if your suspicions are correct.

But can she treat your child? In most cases, the answer is yes, but that's not always your best option. Pediatricians are excellent general internists, but in most cases, they do not have the intimate knowledge of diabetes and children that an endocrinologist has. Nor does a pediatrician have a team of diabetes experts to help you with each aspect of the disease. In addition, a pediatrician usually does not have the time you'll need to speak regularly with her for at least the first few weeks (and even months) of your child's diagnosis.

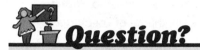

Question?

What if our pediatrician wants to treat our child?
It's kind of your pediatrician to offer but insist that he refer you to a pediatric endocrinologist, even if the endocrinologist is hours away from your home. You'll need the specialized expertise and individualized time that an endocrinologist can offer.

Insurance may restrict where your pediatrician sends you. But if there is a hospital with a pediatric endocrinology center in your general area, expect your pediatrician to help you get referred there.

The Hospital

You'll most likely drive your child to the hospital. If you are too frightened or upset, try to arrange for a family member or good friend to meet you along the way and hop in and drive for you. If your spouse is not nearby, he or she should meet you at the hospital.

Once there, you'll go to the emergency room. In just about every newly diagnosed diabetes case, instead of sitting in the waiting room, you will be jettisoned to a treatment room where your child's health will be assessed. The hospital will be able to get real-time numbers. Most pediatricians' offices have basic meters such as the one you'll use at home that only measure blood sugars up to 500 or so, but hospital labs can get a real number. They'll check ketones right away and also perform tests on other indicators, such as potassium, to determine if your child is in diabetic ketoacidosis (DKA).

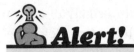

Alert!

While friends and family may want to rush to the emergency room to be by your side, this is no time for a crowd. Ask them to stay home and promise to put one family member in charge of keeping everyone up-to-speed.

Your child will be seen by the attending physician in the emergency room first and will be given an intravenous line right away. The attending physician will then call in the pediatric endocrinology team. They will assess your child, begin the administration of insulin, and take the first steps to help you and your child begin the process of accepting the diagnosis and learning how to live with it. The attending physician and the first endocrinologist will most likely try to soothe you and your child. Many children, particularly those of school age, need to be told that their recent bedwetting and behavior issues were not their fault, and that they are going to be feeling better soon. Parents and caregivers need to be told that insulin works well and that within hours their child will begin feeling better. At that point, parents will start to learn what diabetes means. Some extremely ill children (who are in DKA) may go to intensive care for a day or so, in which case their parents can remain confused and frightened for days.

Outpatient Care

If your child's diagnosis came with a relatively low number and no ketones, you may be sent home and referred to an outpatient learning program the next day. Some parents are frightened by this; the thought of spending a night at home with a child on insulin for the first time is almost too much to bear. Others feel that even after a short outpatient training, they still are not comfortable caring for their child. If this is the case with you, call your pediatrician immediately and tell her how you feel. Ask her to work with you to find an inpatient program, or a better outpatient program, to help you build confidence in your ability to care for your child.

What Happens at the Hospital?

Besides the acute medical intervention your child needs, his hospital stay will also be an immersion class in diabetes care. As stressful and exhausting as an inpatient stay can be, some families prefer them since it gives them medical support to care for their child as they learn how to give shots, how to count carbs, and how to begin to estimate doses.

Stabilizing Your Child

Your hospital medical team will work first and foremost to get your child's blood sugar into an acceptable range and to clear all the ketones from his system. This will mean, at first, insulin and fluids by IV and no food by mouth. Usually, most children (not in an ICU) only need this overnight or for a half day or so. Once the medical team believes your child is within a target range, they will work to get your child off the IV, on to shots, and eating real food again.

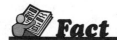 **Fact**

Expect your child to be ravenous at that first meal after diagnosis. Her body has not been metabolizing food for a good long while, and truly eating a meal will be a treat. No need to worry though, your child's appetite will stabilize soon.

Once the team sees your child eating, holding food down, and staying within what will at first be a wide range of target blood glucose readings, your education will begin and so will the transition from the medical team's caring for your child to your doing that on your own. Lean on the team at this time and ask them to help you gain confidence in your skills.

Diabetes 101

Once your child has moved from the emergency room to his inpatient room, a pediatric endocrinologist will begin the process of educating you. Sometimes, particularly if you are in a large city hospital, the endocrinologist is a fellow (a physician who has already completed medical school and preliminary training and is eligible for board certification). Do not let that worry you. If you feel a positive connection, stick with him or her. Fellows are just as dedicated as long-timers and always have the support and oversight of a senior endocrinologist. Many families have stuck with residents for the long haul, celebrating with them when they become attending physicians.

The endocrinologist will describe each member of the team and what the team goals will be for your child (see Chapter 4 for details on who is on your team and how you'll work with them).

The amount of information can be overwhelming. It is important to take notes and keep files right from the start. Ask your spouse or a loved one to get a good organizer (like a loose-leaf notebook with folders that your children use for school) that you can use to keep track of all the new information you'll be given.

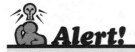

Alert!

Be ready for the first big question your child is going to ask you: "Will I need another shot?" It's inevitable, and you can ask your Certified Diabetes Educator, endocrinologist, or social worker to help you answer that question in a way that is age appropriate for your child.

The first major moment—and one you'll never forget—will be giving your child a shot for the first time. Most hospitals have fake "flabby butts" to practice on; others have you use an orange. It's a good idea to get the feel of a needle's penetration before trying it on your child. Be assured, everyone—even nurses and doctors who give strangers shots all the time—is petrified the first time she gives her own child a shot. It truly is a matter of just doing it. Once you've moved past that first time, you should adapt quickly.

Some older children prefer to give themselves shots from the start. Even so, it's still a good idea for you and your spouse to give a shot or two while at the hospital. You'll need to feel comfortable with the procedure in case your child ever needs help.

Finger pricks, too, are a learned process. You'll want to learn how to choose the best spot on your child's finger and why rotating is important. Again, even if your child chooses to do it alone, insist on doing it a few times yourself while you have educational support there.

 Essential

Forget the bandages on the fingertips. You simply cannot consider finger sticks a boo-boo; like it or not, they will be a part of life. Try to picture your child with a bandage on each of six or more finger pricks a day. It's just not practical.

You'll quickly learn, too, that diabetes does not mean the end of all sugar in your child's diet. Ask your nutritionist to help you create a diet plan that's as close as possible to any child's lifestyle. You may even want to let your child have a treat like a cupcake or candy in the hospital, so she (and you) can see that it can, indeed, be done.

The Emotional Toll

Diagnosis time can be one of the most emotionally challenging times for parents, children, relatives, and even friends. An incurable disease that demands a lifetime of constant care is no easy pill to swallow, particularly when it's your child who has it. Everyone reacts in his own way, but there are common threads and ways of coping.

Parental Guilt

Parents or caregivers can feel guilty at this time, for more than just not seeing the symptoms early enough (because in most cases, almost everyone thinks they took too long). Your medical team should tell you, but if they don't, be assured: You did nothing as a parent to cause this disease, and there was nothing you could do to avoid it.

Because the majority of people with diabetes have Type 2, this disease is often thought to be controllable or even avoidable. Type 1 diabetes is neither. Once that trigger clicked and your child's immune system decided to wreak havoc on her insulin-producing cells, you could not stop it from happening.

Sometimes parents of adopted children will question if there was something in their medical background that could have forewarned them about the diagnosis. The simple answer is no. While children and other relatives of people with Type 1 run a slightly higher risk of developing diabetes, it is still uncommon enough for the disease to be shared by relatives that it is not considered familial.

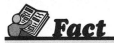 **Fact**

According to a National Institutes of Health study, only about 2.2 percent of children of parents with Type 1 diabetes develop Type 1. However Type 2 diabetes is more likely to develop in someone whose parent, grandparent, or sibling also has the disease.

In other words, medical history or not, you most likely did not give your child diabetes. Ironically, one of the most common questions you'll be asked by friends and even strangers is, "Who gave it to him? You or your wife?" The answer, you can say with all confidence, is neither one. It takes a combination of genetics and environment to cause Type 1 diabetes, and as of yet, no one has discovered what that environmental trigger is.

Feeding your child differently would not have changed his fate either. Too much sugar does not cause diabetes. Some studies have looked at the introduction of cow's milk into a child's diet and the onset of diabetes, but there is no clinical proof that any one thing is a cause.

Parental Fear

Most parents are just plain afraid as well—afraid to give that first shot, afraid to be responsible for their child's well-being, afraid of the future. This is normal, and you should talk about it with your medical team.

The best weapon you'll have to battle your very appropriate parental fear is knowledge. Ask your team about blood sugars and what is safe and unsafe and what is a reason to panic. Talk to them about complications and how the world has changed for the better when it comes to offsetting them and treating them if they do come along. It's going to be vital for you, as a parent, to take your fear, deal with it, and work your way toward understanding and confidence. Long-term parental fear can hurt a child's self-esteem and build panic issues in children as well. Yes, diabetes is scary, but it's nothing you cannot deal with once you have support, education, and a good medical team.

Kids' Guilt and Fear

It will be important, too, to let your child know he did nothing wrong to end up in this position, and that he should always feel comfortable voicing his fears to you. Have a discussion, with the hospital social worker present, about what your child is thinking and feeling. Each age has unique issues and answers. Be sure to build a relationship with the social worker right there in the hospital so that your child has another adult, an expert, whom he can trust to help him deal with his worries and fears. Your child will need this support now and as the years go by.

How and What to Tell Your Friends

Everyone, everyone, is going to want to know what is going on and have an opinion about what they think is going on. While your time needs to be focused on your child and your diabetes skills at this time, finding a way to reach out to friends and family to keep them informed will help make your transition home less bumpy.

Appoint a Spokesperson

No, you're not NASA or the governor, but having a family spokesperson is a great idea at the start. Your friends and family will all want to hear what is going on and how you all are doing. You, however, will be completely immersed in learning all you need to learn. By cutting down the number of people you talk to at certain points during the day, you'll make it easier to focus on what you need to and not leave your well-intentioned friends in the dark.

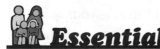 **Essential**

Use technology to keep friends and family up-to-date, too. A nightly e-mail blast sent by your spokesperson or by you if your hospital has Internet access can keep your friends and family in the loop and yet will not be too taxing on your precious time and energy.

Plan on talking to your spokesperson twice a day, and give her an update to pass on ("Joey had Dad do his first shot today and it went really well," or, "The doctors are happy to see that he's reacting well to the first doses of insulin"). This will help keep your friends informed and let them know that you all are safe and relatively well.

Friend Pre-education

Your spokesperson should also encourage your friends and family to begin learning about diabetes and children before you get home. Have your spokesperson direct them to Web sites like jdrf.org and childrenwithdiabetes.com for basics. Ask your medical team for some book suggestions so your friends can read up on the basics. If you don't have to explain the simplest things, you'll have more time to get really meaningful support from your friends.

The Guts to Go Home

More than one parent has felt it: Your child is happy in the activity room, and you're comfortable surrounded by the medical team and their support. True, the parent bed in the hospital room is not so comfortable, and the food is getting boring, but couldn't you just live there from now on? Getting the guts to go home is a major step in working back toward your new "normal" life.

Preparation

Your medical team should make sure you leave the hospital armed not only with information, books, and papers to explain all the details (all of which they've gone over with you) but also with all your prescriptions filled. Most hospitals have a pharmacy. If yours does not, fill your scripts at a nearby one, and then bring them back to your child's room. Going through the actual items with your medical team one more time will help you get acquainted with the tools you will use to help your child stay well.

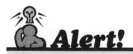

Alert!

Have someone bring a small cooler to the hospital on discharge day. That way, you won't risk your month's supply of insulin getting warm if the car ride ends up extended for any reason.

Parents should also leave the hospital with some level of confidence. You should have given your child a shot at least a couple of times. You should understand how and when to use a glucagon kit; the kit contains a needle and a dose of the hormone glucagon and is used to counteract the seriously low blood sugar levels that cause seizures (see Chapter 6 for more information). You should have a cursory knowledge of carbohydrates and a small booklet, which you can refer to at all times, that lists the amount of carbs found in foods. Finally, you should have the twenty-four-hour emergency phone number for the medical team.

The First Plan

Your child will not go home on the diabetes plan that she will stay on long-term. Your team should sit down with you and come up with temporary target blood glucose ranges as well as an insulin-dosing plan for the first days. Expect that to change quickly, but you can stick by it for the first few days. Expect your child's target range to be a bit higher than you may have read is good (some books call for target ranges from 80 to 140). Newly diagnosed families usually opt, with their team's advice, for something more like 100 to 200 or even higher for tinier tots. As you learn more and become more comfortable, your team will help you pull that target range in tighter. Now, on your way home, is the time to learn to be comfortable, not to shoot for perfect numbers.

In the end, heading home will be the best thing that happens to you. True, you face a whole new world of challenges, but as you face each one, you and your child will find that you can still live happy, active, and normal lives.

Chapter 4

Bonding with Your Diabetes Team

Your pediatric endocrinology team will become your touch point, sometimes even your lifesaver. Finding a quality team, knowing what to expect from them, and understanding the role each member of the team plays will be key to your success as the parent or caregiver of a child with diabetes. This chapter will introduce you to the major players on your child's medical team and provide insights into finding the right people for you and your child to work with.

The Pediatric Endocrinologist

It takes a special kind of human to have the dedication, knowledge, and sensitivity required to be a pediatric endocrinologist. As you probably realize by now, children with diabetes and their families are among the neediest (for good reason) patient groups that exist. A good pediatric endocrinologist takes the time to know his or her patients (and families) personally, to weigh in on important issues, and to be up-to-date on treatment. A good patient family knows how to use that dedication and not abuse it.

The Endocrinologist's Job

Your endocrinologist should be your team leader, coming second only to you when it comes to the over-all well-being of your child. Although you won't meet with or talk to her about everything, she should be

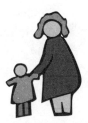

up-to-date and informed on everything that's going on in your child's life with diabetes. When it comes to your child's care and your endocrinologist, you should expect her to look at the entire care program and how the child is progressing, not necessarily minute details.

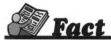 **Fact**

The first official pediatric endocrinologist is thought to be Lawson Wilkins (1894–1963). He created the specialization while working at Johns Hopkins Medical School in the 1940s. Dr. Wilkins started a clinic devoted to pediatric endocrinology and focused on the problems of growth and genetics.

It is important for parents (and patients) to remember that while they'd like to think they are their endocrinologist's only patients, they are not. At the same time, a patient should never feel put off or ignored. The balance should come from the family's understanding that the endocrinologist is an overseer and the endocrinologist's commitment to seeing the child at least twice a year and to being willing to have a phone discussion almost any time.

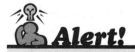 **Alert!**

Children with diabetes can be at a higher risk for other endocrine disorders, such as thyroid disease and celiac disease. Your endocrinologist should always be on the lookout for signs of other disorders, but he should do so in a way that doesn't cause panic to you or your child.

A bonus is that some pediatric endocrinologists are involved in research as well. Imagine that your child's physician could be the one who finds the cure for diabetes, or even is in on a treatment breakthrough. It can be exciting and motivating to hear up-to-date research news from your endocrinologist from time to time.

Hunting Them Down

For families near big cities, finding a good pediatric endocrinologist can be as simple as phoning the major teaching and children's hospitals in your area (see Appendix B for more details). You may also want to ask other families about their experiences. Remember, though, it's kind of like teachers: One child and family may click with a certain endocrinologist that another does not. It's a personal experience, and you'll need, in the end, to judge for yourself what works best for you.

For families who live in rural areas, finding a good pediatric endocrinologist can be a treasure hunt.

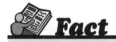 *Fact*

According to *Endocrine Today* magazine, only twenty-six states have at least one pediatric endocrinologist per 100,000 children and two states—Wyoming and Montana—have none. You will need to do your research and rely on your pediatrician for help.

"Treasure hunt" is an apt term because a quality pediatric endocrinologist is worth searching for and driving a distance to visit. If you live in a rural area, you may need to depend on a general pediatrician for most things, but every family should have a medical team headed by a certified pediatric endocrinologist caring for their child, even if it means fewer appointments and more frequent telephone and e-mail consultations. The endocrinologist is the co-captain you need to win this battle.

The Certified Diabetes Educator (CDE)

Every good pediatric endocrinology team has a Certified Diabetes Educator. Though they are most often nurses, CDEs can also come from other specialties such as nutrition and physiology. Shoot for the best scenario: a nurse who is trained as a CDE. (CDEs, by the way, must recertify every five years, keeping them up-to-date on the ever-changing diabetes care landscape.) Your CDE will, from the start, be your navigator, teacher, and support person through the nuts and bolts of life with diabetes.

A good CDE helps move you and your child, at the pace that works best for you, from being completely cared for with full support to being able to live with the disease with lesser support. Expect to have appointments with your CDE at least twice a year (usually rotating with the pediatric endocrinologist's appointments). CDEs are usually adept as well at helping you consider new therapies such as different insulin and equipment like insulin pumps.

The CDE's Job

While the endocrinologist is about the big picture, the CDE fills in the pieces and connects the dots. Think of the CDE as your child's life coach in diabetes. A good CDE knows how to guide a family through the day-to-day challenges of life with diabetes, at every age. More important, a good CDE knows how to empower a family and child to work through those challenges.

 Essential

Your child's bond with his CDE may be the most important one he forms. If he does not seem to get along well with or respect his current CDE, ask your endocrinologist to help you make a change. If there is only one choice, talk to the CDE about the situation.

Look to your CDE to teach you basics such as how to give injections and how to keep a logbook. These specialists are often the ones to help you figure out which insulin you might want your child to use and how to plan for special events and changes in life. They are usually up-to-speed on meters and technology and can help you pick new items when you are looking for a change.

With the advent of pumps and kids (remember, less than a decade ago, few children were on pumps), the job of helping families decide on whether pumping is the right choice and then starting the process usually falls to the CDE. Some large diabetes centers even have CDEs whose sole job is to get a child up and running on an insulin pump. (For more on pump technology, see Chapter 7.)

CDEs and Support

From the start, families and children tend to lean heavily on their CDEs for help and support. This is natural. The CDE is your shoulder in the hospital, your teacher in the first weeks, and your point of reference in times of question.

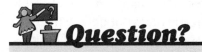 **Question?**

Can my child's caretaker be my friend too?
So close and intense is the relationship between CDEs or endocrinologists and parents or caregivers that often, friendship blossoms. This is a great situation. Just remember, like teachers, there are professional lines that should never be crossed and that can make friendships rough at times.

Certified Diabetes Educators should be knowledgeable about support programs in your area and about online support as well. If you've had a hard time and are feeling alone, although you'd love to ask your CDE just to move into your house already, it's better to just let her know how you are feeling and ask her to point you toward support.

The Nutritionist

Your nutritionist, or registered dietitian, will be your guide for all that is food in your first months and even years. Although there will come a time when you'll know just about everything and your appointments with your nutritionist will feel more like catching up with an old friend, you should plan on having your child visit with him, in the long run, at least annually. Food likes and dislikes change, as does a child's metabolism. There's always something to tweak, and the nutritionist is the one to tweak it.

Meal Plans or Not?

Not long ago, all children newly diagnosed with diabetes went immediately on a meal plan. It was pretty much cast in stone, and it represented all the food groups. Basically, it was a low-sugar, moderate-fat diet. While no one debates that is the best way for a child with diabetes to eat, nutritionists who work with kids with diabetes are quick to point out that the most important thing you can do with a diet is make a child feel like a *child* and not like a victim.

For that reason, some nutritionists are willing to be more flexible. Most nutritionists will be willing to help you and your child work out a flexible plan that helps you live a more normal lifestyle. Still, in a perfect plan, meals should be carefully timed in all cases. For instance, if a snack is too close to a dinnertime check, blood glucoses can be falsely high, since insulin would still be working on them.

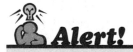

Alert!

Foods metabolize differently in every child. Don't take a diabetes friend's word for how to cover a certain food with insulin. Though this friend may have experience, he is not a medical professional. Rather, talk to your nutritionist about a plan that is tailor-made for that food and your child.

Even with flexibility, though, it's a good idea to let a nutritionist come up with a series of meal plans for your child. Use these plans as best you can, since, as every diabetes caregiver eventually realizes, repetition is the key to success. (Some famed athletes with Type 1 say their secret to success is eating the exact same foods at the exact same time every day.) Use the plans as a starting point, and ask your nutritionist to help you figure out how to deviate for special occasions, parties, or just because you feel like it.

Label Language

A good nutritionist will also help you become a label translator. Ask your nutritionist to allow you to bring the labels of some of your child's favorite foods and help you to understand what all the ingredients mean. Ask her to help you understand things like glycemic indexing and whether "sugar alcohols" count. In time, your nutritionist should have you speaking the same language she speaks, and understanding, for the most part, what foods mean to your child's diabetes.

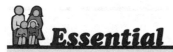

Essential

Eventually, as your child grows, work toward a time when your nutritionist meets alone with your child, at least for part of the appointment. This will help shift the responsibility of understanding foods to your child, something that once he is fully grown must become a reality.

A nutritionist can also help fill in the blanks for the rest of the team on other issues. The nutritionist may pick up on signs of a possible eating disorder or other type or problem; the kind of information that, shared with the rest of the team, could help your child avoid a crisis or recover quickly from one.

The Social Worker

Although every good medical team has a social worker on board, the social worker tends to be the team member families know least as time goes on. This is ironic because your social worker can be a gold mine of support, ideas, and information at every stage of your child's life with diabetes.

Remove the Stigma

Every family should meet with the team social worker at diagnosis time, whether it's in the hospital or as an outpatient. At that time, the social worker will be assessing your family to see if there are any special needs. Social workers have an excellent general knowledge in areas like making your insurance work for you, setting up a program in school that works for your child, and understanding the psychological ramifications of the onset of diabetes on the patient and the entire family.

 Essential

Chances are you won't have actual appointments with your social worker. Ask her, ahead of time, to pop in and say hi at all of your endocrinologist appointments for the first year. This way, you'll all get to know one another before a crisis call is needed.

By making the social worker another nice person your child knows on the medical team, you'll help remove any feelings of shame that your child might have if and when the time comes that you feel a full appointment with a social worker is needed.

How a Social Worker Can Help

The social worker is trained to help you cope with any unusual situations that may arise in your life with diabetes. A small child heads home from the hospital after diagnosis and begins sleeping in his parent's room again every night. What's a family to think or do? Your social worker can give you insight. A teenager who has been compliant for years suddenly refuses to care for herself (see Chapter 16 for more on teen issues). Your social worker can intervene and give you excellent insights and also help you find the perfect therapist, should you agree your child needs one.

How to Find a Good Match

Everyone in the diabetes world has their own opinion on pediatric endocrinologists. Who's good? Who's bad? Who cares? Who should be avoided? The best thing you can do when selecting a team is simple: Don't take anyone else's opinions to heart. Choosing a good team is rather like choosing a good teacher or even a good mate. Everyone has their own quirks, their own likes and dislikes. Most parents or caregivers have had that experience when another parent tells them to steer clear of a certain teacher, only to have their child adore that teacher. Relationships are subjective and organic. Trusting your instincts will make a difference.

The Search

Some families are lucky; the endocrinology team that treats their child in the hospital at diagnosis just feels right. If this is the case, you've hit the jackpot. Even if other well-intentioned folks try to tell you that the best place is somewhere else, go with your gut and let this relationship continue.

If your child was not treated in a place with a full pediatric endocrinology team, you'll need to begin your search immediately. How do you find one? Although the Web offers you lists and locations at the touch of a key, you'll need to do more than that. First, set your standards.

Keep in mind here that you are the employer and that the team is, for the sake of simplicity, employed by you. Don't hesitate to ask any questions that come to mind before choosing a team.

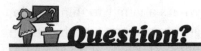 *Question?*

What if the endocrinologist we like is a student?
Stick with her. All pediatric endocrinologist fellows are supported by attending doctors, and often, children click well with young hip students. Many families stick with fellows through their entire education and continue with them when they become attending physicians.

Questions may include but are not limited to the following:

- How often will the pediatric endocrinologist personally see my child?
- Is the support staff, such as the nutritionist and social worker, on site?
- If the team is not at a hospital setting, what hospital affiliation do they have?
- Does the team have live support available twenty-four hours a day?
- What percentage of their patients has Type 1?

Asking these questions will help you get a general feel for what type of program it is and what type of support you can expect. In the beginning, be picky. For instance, if you are the type of parent who wants the endocrinologist herself to see your child at least twice a year, do not settle for a team that has your child meet always with the Certified Diabetes Educator. If you'll only feel comfortable with a team that answers calls twenty-four hours a day (and does not rely on an answering service that can leave you hanging for hours), keep searching until you find one, or until you've exhausted all options.

What's in a Name?

There are well-known names in every city that leave diabetes patients in awe. But a big name does not always mean it's your only smart choice. History can mean a lot in diabetes care, and you should pay attention to that. But a name itself does not make a quality program. Even when dealing with the most famous names, ask all the obvious questions. If you find a smaller, lesser-known pediatric diabetes program that offers everything you want and feels like the place for you, ignore the well-intentioned friends who will say things like, "Surely you're going to the Big Name Here center. Why would you go anywhere else?"

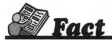 **Fact**

One good bonus to a program name that includes a hospital name is simple. Should your child ever be hospitalized, she'll be treated by the same team of doctors and nurses that treats her as an outpatient. There is value in that familiar situation.

Like everything else in diabetes and children, you know best what is right for you and your family. Trust your decisions. And remember, you can always change if you are unhappy or if circumstances change.

Building a Positive Relationship

Like any important, long-term relationship in your life, the one you have with your child's medical team will need attention, care, and some give-and-take. Making sure your expectations are clear and your mind is kept open will pave the way to great care for your child.

Who's the Boss?

You are. But then again, it's not that simple. It is vital for parents or caregivers of children with diabetes (as it is for parents or caregivers of children with any disease) to feel empowered. No one, even the most dedicated doctor on earth, cares more for your child and his future than you do. It's fine to embrace that and remind everyone of that. Any time it comes down to push versus shove, you will always have the final say.

That being said, a good boss knows how to delegate responsibility and use the insight of trusted experts around him. This situation is no different. You need to have a healthy respect for each member of your team. Because although parents often do become just about as close to a fully trained, unlicensed endocrinologist as someone can get, your pediatric endocrinologist is still the trained doctor. If she tells you that you're running your child's blood sugars too low, take what she is saying into consideration. Ask for backup information. Debate, but don't argue.

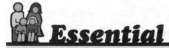 **Essential**

Often, new technology is pushed more by patient families than by staff. If you find a new tool you'd like to see your team begin using, ask them to consider meeting with the tool's representatives. Don't assume you need to go elsewhere to use a new tool.

Some parents might find it intimidating to debate with a doctor; you simply cannot afford to be intimidated. As long as you are respectful and listen to the doctor's side, fight for whatever care you think your child needs.

When to Call and When Not to Call

It's easy to get addicted to calling your medical team for advice. It's just as easy to feel guilty and not call often enough. Knowing when to call and what to call about will help show your team that you understand and respect them. When you call for the right reasons, they should always welcome your call.

If your child's blood sugar does something that concerns you (such as a violent swing upward or downward that you do not understand), it is always okay to phone the doctor on call. Even if all they say is "It's fine," it is always better to err on the side of caution, and your team understands that. Usually, in the first months, parents make a lot of these calls. As time goes on and you begin to trust your own actions and reactions to highs and lows, you'll eventually find you really don't need to call for that reason as much.

If your child has unexplained ketones or large ketones at any time, it is always right to call. Ketones are always an emergency situation (see Chapter 19 for more details on sick day management), and parents often need a doctor or nurse to talk them through the process of bringing that blood sugar down.

If your child is vomiting, a call to the team is always warranted. (Again, see Chapter 19 for details.)

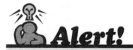

Alert!

Never depend on e-mail communication for an emergency medical situation. E-mail and wireless communication may seem real-time solutions, but voice-to-voice contact is the only option in an emergency situation.

It's not okay to telephone a doctor who is on call in the middle of the night for a prescription refill. Unless you've dropped all your insulin on the floor in the middle of the night, maintenance things like script refills should always be handled with calls during regular office hours. So, too, should appointment cancellations. Silly as it sounds, some parents do telephone on-call doctors for such things.

On the other hand, any time you are at your wit's end and you need to talk to an expert immediately, your team should respect that, as silly as your need may seem later. Both sides need to have compassion, patience, and some give-and-take. With that, a good team will help your child until the cure is found.

CHAPTER 5

Letters, Numbers, and Other Diabetes Codes

W hen you first hear it, it's like some kind of secret agent code. The terms, abbreviations, and details of Type 1 diabetes are almost a mystery to outsiders. As hard as it is to remember at the start if your child has Type 1 or Type 2 (or was that Type A or Type B?), there's more code to crack, concepts to understand, and ways to keep in tune with what is going on with your child's diabetes.

DKA

These three letters strike fear into the heart of anyone dealing with Type 1 diabetes. Shorthand for *diabetic ketoacidosis*, DKA is a serious and life-threatening condition in which the body is so deprived of insulin that the patient can lapse into a coma and even die. Understanding what DKA is, what causes it, and how to avoid it is crucial in diabetes care.

What Is It?

Diabetic ketoacidosis is a condition in which the body is so deprived of insulin that it becomes desperate for fuel and begins breaking down fatty tissue and muscle. Ketones are the by-product of this process, and the liver can only process a certain amount of ketones at a time. When the body produces too many ketones, they spill over into the bloodstream and, like an acid, basically

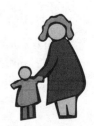

poison the person. This process also results in a lack of bicarbonate, as well as other lab abnormalities that your medical or ER team will look for in your child at presentation. Symptoms include frequent urination, dehydration, excessive thirst, and sometimes stomach pain and even some cramping. Vomiting often occurs as well.

Causes of DKA

The cause is, put simply, a lack of insulin in the body. But how that lack of insulin comes to be can be more complicated. At diagnosis, DKA is usually because parents and/or the patient did not know the signs of the onset of diabetes, and the patient hovered at a high blood glucose number for an extended period.

Well into treatment, DKA can be caused by a massive infection or major illness and sometimes by a malfunctioning pump or site. In some cases, particularly with teens and adults, DKA can be caused by the purposeful withholding of insulin. Sometimes, teens with diabetes don't take insulin so they'll lose weight quickly. Other times, teens stop caring for themselves because they are sick of the lifestyle diabetes has forced on them.

It can be tough for a parent or caregiver to notice DKA the first time, particularly if a child is handing all her own care. By seeing your child's meter at least a few times a day, you may help avoid DKA.

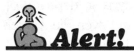

Alert!

Diabetic ketoacidosis is a true emergency. If you suspect it, call your medical team immediately and plan on heading to the emergency room. You need hands-on professional help to correct the situation.

This condition doesn't always occur as a result of high blood sugars. Some children struggle with ketones when they have a stomach bug or other kind of vomiting situation. If your child is vomiting, you absolutely need to check regularly for ketones, no matter what his blood sugar reading is. It is possible to be low and have a large number of ketones, a situation that needs medical intervention as well.

How to Avoid DKA

The best way to avoid DKA is to be vigilant about checking for ketones. Although it's driven into the minds of most parents at diagnosis time, many parents cease checking for ketones every time a blood sugar reading is over 260, because they understand the reason a child is high and feel confident they know how to correct the situation.

But in reality, the best-care scenario always includes checking for ketones when a child's reading is over 260, or when a child is experiencing any kind of illness.

It's also important to remember that when ketones are present, the correction factor is higher. You'll want to talk to your medical team ahead of time about what they'd like you to do when ketones are present (many will give a percentage increase for you to go by; others will ask you always to call for help with ketones). Either way, the first couple of times you'll want to call for help just to gain confidence.

Avoiding DKA can come with vigilance and oversight as well. If you look at your child's meter at least three times a day, she won't have enough time to slip into DKA without you knowing.

Public Shame

Some parents feel ashamed after their child is diagnosed with DKA. It's a prideful thing, caring for your child with diabetes. But remember, we are all human. Some parents also experience grief after a DKA incident, almost like the feeling at diagnosis time. Talk to your social worker if you experience grief or shame. He or she will help you see that you are not alone.

A1c—It's Not as Easy as ABC

The A1c—or your child's three-month average blood sugar—quickly becomes a number you live by. It has many nicknames, such as hemoglobin A1c, HbA1c, glycohemoglobin, glycolated hemoglobin, and glycosylated hemoglobin. Parents need to understand not only what the A1c means, but also how to use that information to help their child.

What Is the A1c?

The A1c is a big picture of how in or out of range your child's blood glucose levels are over an extended period. A1c numbers differ from blood glucose numbers. Lab normal (in most labs) for a person without diabetes is 4.1–6.1 percent. To get an idea of what A1cs translate to, an A1c of 6 percent equals average blood glucose of about 135. You can add 30 to that number for every 1 percent increase in A1c, giving you an idea of what your child's true average is. Because meter checks only represent a brief moment in time, the A1c average may differ from what you are seeing on your meter.

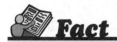 **Fact**

Expect your child to have an A1c drawn at least four times a year. Ask your medical team if this will be the case for your child, and if it is not, ask that it be so from this time on. Be assertive for your child and proactive in her goal of a healthy lifestyle.

For very young children, medical teams often set a higher goal range for A1c levels, since the risk of lows can be greater with a small child who cannot recognize symptoms. For older children and adults, the tighter you keep your diabetes in control, the less chance of complications later in life. So target ranges are often aggressive. The American Diabetes Association recommends that every person with Type 1 should try to keep his or her level below 7. This is not easy to do, and your medical team won't want you and your child to beat yourselves up over it. Talk to them about the range they'd like to see your child in, and ways you can work to get there.

How to Make the A1c Work for You

It's easy to fall into a trap with A1cs. For many parents, they're almost like the SATs. While parents should be careful never to call their children's blood glucose readings "tests," some look toward the A1c as if it were a midterm exam. They feel as if they're being graded. It's hard not to feel this way. But passing that feeling on to your child can have consequences. Find a way to simply use the A1c as information, not as judgment.

Spikes in A1c Levels

A sudden spike in an A1c level is a reason for concern. Your child may have completely outgrown her dosages and need a new plan. Or, your child could be withholding insulin without your knowing it. Even if your child is still in the 7s but has gone up a full percentage point, it's time to sit down and study the situation to determine what is changing, so adjustments can be made. This is exactly what the A1c is for: helping and guiding, not judging. Remember, if some boastful parent roughs you up by bragging about her child's 5.2 A1c, keep in mind that parents lie about A1cs just as they do about SATs. Take it with a grain of salt. Also keep in mind that some doctors advise against too low an A1c level in children because it can make feeling blood sugar lows more difficult. Come up with a personal plan for your child and forget everyone else.

Breaking Down Daily Averages

As you progress as a diabetes parent, you'll learn to look not just at the A1c and meter average but also at averages for each time of day. You'll learn what times of day to study and what to do with the information you get to help your child maintain better control.

Rise and Shine

Morning numbers are the foundation of a well-controlled diabetes day. If you can work to get your child waking up in a range you and your team agree is a good one for him, you'll be a step closer to tight control. But mornings can be tricky. There's the entire night that needs to be handled (and no parent wants to check a child two or three times each night), and many people with diabetes experience a spike in blood sugars as the sun rises. This is usually caused by something called the "dawn phenomenon."

The dawn phenomenon can cause blood sugar to rise, since the body needs an extra boost of insulin at that time. Kids on pumps can up their basal rate for those few hours; kids on shots will need to figure out which insulin should be increased so it peaks to match the glucose surge.

Fret not: This does not mean you'll need to be up all night every night for the rest of your child's life. But it does mean you'll be doing numerous night checks for an entire night from time to time. In an ideal world, you'd do checks every two hours through the night once every six weeks or so to gather the information you and your team need to make changes to help get that morning glucose reading in target range.

You may find, with that checking, that your child's morning high is not from dawn phenomenon, but actually from something called the Somogyi effect, which is a rebound high after a nighttime low. If this is the case, ask your team to help you adjust for less insulin earlier at night instead.

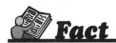 **Fact**

Even people without diabetes have the "dawn phenomenon." Because hormones that work against insulin production surge in the predawn hours, people without diabetes have increased insulin production at that time.

Midday Readings

Throughout the day, you'll want to know how your child reacts to meals. This is why in addition to lunch and snack time readings, postprandial readings are helpful as well. Postprandial readings, taken about an hour and a half to two hours after a meal or snack, show you if the insulin you gave for that food covered it well.

These readings will also help you find out which foods react differently in your child. You may find that pasta or pizza keeps her blood sugar high longer, so you can change the insulin dose based on that information.

Of course, checking a child at every meal and at every postprandial may be too much. Instead, focus on one meal time at a time and do postprandial for it for a week, watching for a pattern. Then move on to another meal. If you keep good records, you should be able to gather enough data to last a good long time.

Bedtime

What's the best number for a child who is ready to go to sleep? The answer varies from child to child and depends on what kind of insulin therapy you are using. If your child is pumping, you'll be able to set basals to vary through the night. If your child is still on a peaking insulin, you may want to talk to your team about what number is safe for bedtime.

But even when you've found the right number, you'll need to know your child is safe all night long. While some children wake up when they feel high or low, others do not. Plan on checking your child at your bedtime as well (if you stay up later than she does), and set a goal of a middle-of-the-night check at least once a week. If your spouse can do one as well, that would be two a week with each of you only having to get up once. This should be enough information to keep your child safe. Some parents argue that middle-of-the-night checks are needed each night. That decision is up to you and your team.

If your child gets up more than once to go to the bathroom at night, you may want to do a quick check as well, since increased urination can be a sign of high blood sugar. Of course, there will come the day that your child says, "But Dad! Everyone pees!" and she's right. But checking means better safe than sorry, and one more number gives you more data to work with, leading you to in-target averages.

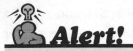

Alert!

Nighttime lows can be caused by the level your child drops to and also by how far that drop is. So if you put a child to bed with a high number, you'll want to check him in two hours or so to make sure he's feeling okay and his number is within range.

Realistic Goals at All Ages

Okay, so you want your child to be between 80 and 130 and have an A1c of 6.2 at all times. Don't all parents of diabetic children? But in reality, goals change with age. A realistic goal set by you and your medical team will help your child grow up healthy, both physically and emotionally.

Little Ones

For many reasons, target glucose levels need to be adapted for little ones. Usually, a goal range is about 100–200 for toddlers, pre-schoolers, and even young elementary-school kids. There are a few reasons for this target range. First, it's harder for little ones to feel lows and highs coming on. Tighter control means more of a risk for lows, and having a higher low range can help avoid that. You may read that the ideal range is 80 to 130, but that is not the case here. Keeping a target range like that at this age is completely appropriate, and as your medical team will tell you, it is healthy for your child.

Elementary School Through Junior High

These are the years your children want to please you, and a tighter goal can be reached. Kids this age tend to be (for the most part) compliant and obedient; they are usually not against public displays of their diabetes. This is an age when you can ask your child to check more often and keep tighter control. But don't take it too far. You don't want to push burnout.

Keep in mind, too, that you may want to change your goals for special days, such as sports days or extra active days. Even with compliant kids, lows can come fast on unusually active days. So cutting off at 100 or even 120 on those days can be a good idea.

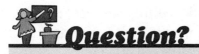 **Question?**

How often is too often to check blood sugars?
The answer to that should come from your child. There's a minimum they have to check (and your team will help decide that); beyond that, let your child be open about what he is willing to do. And respect his decision.

High School Kids

As will be discussed in Chapter 18, high school is a challenging time. Although your ultimate goal needs to be a tight target range, that may take some compromise. Look for your medical team to help you help your teen feel as if she is choosing the target range. Hope for personal buy-in. And if worse comes to worse, set goals one day at a time. Remember too that teens are quite active socially, and you may want to set different goals for driving or all-night parties such as the prom.

Good Numbers Versus Bad Numbers

It's easy for parents and caregivers to begin seeing numbers as good and bad, when in reality, numbers simply provide useful information for you to use to make decisions. It will take time to train yourself not to think of numbers in terms of good or bad.

The "Good" Trap

Diabetes parents are big reward givers because they often feel they have to make up for the bad hand their child was dealt. So a trip to the endocrinologist or the blood lab often involves stopping off for a balloon, a toy, or a special meal. There's nothing wrong with that, just as long as it doesn't go too far.

A child should never be rewarded for having what you see as "good" numbers or a "good" A1c. This is not because she doesn't deserve it; she does. But once you set up that something is good and deserves a reward, you've also introduced the converse, meaning some numbers, in your child's mind, might be bad or deserving of punishment. This is not healthy for a child's self-esteem.

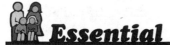

Essential

You can occasionally use bribery as a tool. For example, say your teen asks if he can have a video iPod if he gets his A1c down to the 7s. It's okay to say yes to this deal. If he does not get his numbers down, don't call it failure; it's just a delay in success since the bribe will remain available.

Parents who never say good or bad can often discover they've projected it nonetheless, and that's only human too. A 500 blood sugar reading can be frightening, and so can a 30. Try to reach the point of being able to remain calm in front of your child about her numbers. React calmly and efficiently. Find another place and time, away from your child, to express your fear. You don't want to scare her when it really does not help.

The "Bad" Trap

Admit it: You've been angry about a blood sugar, an A1c, or a pattern you see in your child's care. Diabetes is frustrating, not just to the child but to the parent as well. Getting upset is natural, but it doesn't help the situation. If you ever go over the edge, as soon as you pull yourself together, apologize to your child and explain that you were stressed and should not have been. Let him know you respect his efforts and say it out loud again: Every number is a good number, because it gives you useful information.

You'll need to ask others to avoid the bad trap as well. In general, people like to say things like "Oh, that child is noncompliant," or even, "he's a bad diabetic." Remind everyone—friends, teachers, school nurses—that they cannot speak in negative terms to your child or about your child when it comes to diabetes.

The Numbers in Your Child's Future

What about the statistics and averages your child will encounter? It's important to be honest, but it's also important to make sure you have the facts before sharing them with your child at any time.

Old Versus New

The long-term prognosis for kids growing up with diabetes has come a long way. Even so, there are still some numbers that may frighten even the most mature child. She may hear that the average lifespan of a child with diabetes is fifteen years less than her contemporaries. This was once true, and with poor control could be today. But your child should know that with effort, tools, and a long-term run at control, that won't pertain to her.

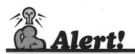

Alert!

There is no need for smaller children to hear any of the speculations or statistics about complications or the dangers they could face as an adult. Let your medical team guide you to the right time and place for your child to hear any of this information.

Your child may also hear that "90 percent of children with diabetes have eye damage as adults." Again, times have changed. When you take your child for his annual eye exam, explain that you have to watch his eyes carefully not because of possible vision loss, but because so many good treatments are available now that your eye doctor will make sure your child remains fine.

It's a Long Road

It is important to stress to your child, too, that she has a long life to work at controlling numbers, and over the years, it's the long run that matters. Point out how far daily care has come, and let her know that many better options are on the horizon. Reassure her that one short period of higher numbers is not the end of the world, and that the future is bright.

CHAPTER 6
Tools of the Trade

Mastering diabetes in the twenty-first century is as much about mastering technology as it is about understanding physiology. In the past two decades, diabetes technology has flourished, and it continues to do so. Parents who learn which tools are best for their child and become proficient in using them find that life with diabetes is a whole lot easier than it might be otherwise.

The Way It Used to Be

In the grand scheme of things, insulin itself is a relatively new medicine. Invented in 1923 by the team of Frederick Banting and Charles Best in Canada, insulin was an instant miracle. Before its invention, children who were diagnosed with Type 1 diabetes slowly (and sometimes not so slowly) starved to death. The only option open to parents was to bring their children with diabetes to special in-patient clinics where they were kept on very low calorie diets, the thought being the less sugar a child's body had to process, the longer he could live with diabetes. The longest a child usually lasted, even in these horrific conditions, was about two years.

Essential

A must-read for parents of children with diabetes is *The Discovery of Insulin* by Michael Bliss. The book traces the treatment of diabetes before insulin, the groundbreaking work of Banting and Best, the delivery of insulin to the marketplace, and the controversy surrounding who received credit for the discovery.

Once insulin was available, the way diabetes was viewed changed instantly. Rather than a quick death sentence, diabetes became something a child could live with. Parents were then faced with the reality of raising a child with a chronic, incurable disease. Although this was clearly a miraculous choice considering that just a handful of years earlier their child would have died, it created its own challenges. Needles were large, painful, and reusable, causing children to develop sores at injection sites. There was no real understanding of how to track blood sugars or what to do about them. Food intake was still strictly monitored and enforced (sugar was a no-no).

Insulin was keeping kids alive. However, because there was only one kind of long-acting insulin and no way to measure blood sugar on a regular basis, the disease still had a severe impact on any life: Frequent lows and highs, erratic blood sugar levels, and complications such as kidney failure and blindness were the norm.

Slow Progress and a Few Clues

As children lived with diabetes and doctors studied the patterns of the disease, they began to realize some facts. Children whose parents worked to keep blood sugars in control as much as possible lived longer and healthier. Most of the Type 1 patients who have received the Eli Lilly Award for living fifty years or more with diabetes recall parents who worked diligently to keep them in some kind of stable range, even without the tools available today. Some parents served smaller meals all day to match the peaks they could see in insulin in the body (just from watching their child's daily patterns). Others painstakingly gathered urine regularly to dip it to check glucose levels. While they didn't have the tools or the know-how yet, these pioneering parents were laying the groundwork for what today is called "tight control."

Most parents now marvel at these stories. As tough as it is today, it's hard to imagine how tough it was, even as recently as the early 1980s.

Today's Insulin Choices

Today's parents have enough insulin choices to create, along with their medical team, a tailor-made insulin care program for their child. But this increase in the number of brands and types was no overnight phenomenon; it was a gradual development that took several years.

New Markets Make Life Better

The first insulin offered to the public was similar to "regular" insulin today. It was short acting—from six to eight hours—and most patients took two or more shots daily and limited calories and carbs to help keep blood sugars down. Then, in 1946 in Denmark, Novo Nordisk debuted NPH insulin, the first long-acting or "cloudy" insulin. NPH, still used in some patients today, works for up to eighteen hours and peaks a number of times during the day. Until quite recently, most Type 1 patients existed on a combination of regular (clear) and NPH (cloudy), taking NPH two times a day and regular insulin two to three times daily and working to create a meal plan that met the many "peaks" in insulin that came with the combination of the two.

A third, even longer-acting insulin usually called Ultralente was put on the market next. The creation of this insulin led NPH to be known as intermediate-acting insulin since the others were longer acting. Ultralente lasts even longer than NPH. Some patients found that using Ultralente and regular insulin, or even all three, worked well over a period lasting twenty-four to thirty-hours.

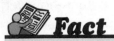 **Fact**

The first patient treated with insulin was Leonard Thompson. In 1922, he was fourteen years old, weighed just sixty-five pounds, and was near death. With insulin, he lived another thirteen years before dying of complications from the disease.

Until just before the twenty-first century, this remained the standard of care for Type 1 patients. With the NPH and regular regime, parents injected their child twice daily with NPH, and in the morning and at dinnertime with regular insulin. The regular insulin did not begin working until a half hour after injection time, so parents injected their children, asked them to wait a half hour, and then expected them to eat exactly the amount of food they'd been injected for. This was a challenging routine particularly for toddlers and small (and sometime rebellious) children. Parents injected their tiny ones and laid out a perfectly planned meal, only to have the tot say, "Me no hungry!" as the regular insulin was beginning to peak.

Quick-Acting Insulin to the Rescue
Needless to say, the advent of super fast-acting insulin such as Humalog and Novolog around 1999 to 2000 was a welcome change. With rapid-acting insulin choices, parents could give their children more freedom, allowing them to eat at less restricted times and to choose the amount of carbs they ate at each meal. In addition, by giving children half a shot at the beginning of a meal and then following up with the balance needed, parents could now allow their children not to finish a planned meal. To parents who had been force-feeding their little ones on regular insulin, this was miraculous.

Around the beginning of the twenty-first century, another insulin was introduced that further modernized insulin therapy. Called Lantus, or insulin glargine, it was a medical breakthrough that stayed working in the body, without peaks, for a full twenty-four hours. Parents who were not ready or interested in an insulin pump found that by using Lantus along with fast-acting insulin for meals, they could mimic a pump without using one. Unlike NPH or Ultralente, this long-acting insulin has no peaks that need to be matched with food.

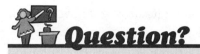 *Question?*

What if my newly diagnosed child is on regular insulin and NPH?
Talk to your medical team about the use of rapid-acting insulin. Ask them to consider letting you put your child on this more flexible, more humane insulin. If they say no, ask for an explanation, and do not rest until they give you one that makes sense.

How to Know What's Best for Your Child

As you mature in your role of a parent of a child with diabetes, you'll begin to wonder about different treatment plans, and you may find one that you feel is right for your child and your family. Knowing which is best and then working on making it happen with your medical team takes education and persuasion.

Family Patterns
First, you need to look at your family patterns. Are you the kind of family that always eats at the same time, has scheduled activities, and sticks to the same routine day in and day out? If so, you may not mind having insulin that peaks multiple times during the day. Some parents find that being forced on to a meal plan because of insulin peaks makes food choices (and demands) easier to follow.

Are you a family that's more seat-of-the-pants? Perhaps you wake up on a Saturday morning and decide, right then, that you want to go hike a mountain ridge you've long eyed. Does your family tend to eat at different times each day? Are you on the run? If this is you, longer-acting insulin with no peaks may be your best choice.

Listen to Your Child

What about your child's opinion? Even the smallest of children can have a say in what type of insulin they end up using. While a child cannot study peak patterns and side effects, she can voice how she feels about her daily routine from a young age.

Ask your preschooler if he likes having a snack two to three times a day and eating on a schedule as NPH requires. Some will say yes; others might say they'd like to be able to eat or not eat when they choose. If your child asks for a different pattern than you've been using, look into an insulin change and when you can make it happen, let her know you listened to her and acted on her wishes.

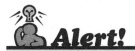

Alert!

Any way you can make your child feel empowered in his medical choices, do it. Kids—even little ones—need to feel they have some control over this disease. Discuss all the options, all the pros and cons of each option with your child, and then come up with a solution together that you both support.

Some children may not like the added daily shots from fast-acting insulin. If you talk to your child about the freedom to eat or not eat when they want and do not plan on going to a pump, you need to explain to her that this will most likely mean more shots. But explain, too, that shots can come in the form of the basic needles she is used to or from insulin pens. Some kids prefer the pens because they can look "cooler and friendlier" and some of the needles might hurt less.

Once you and your child agree on a wanted change, talk to your team. In most cases, if you show them you've done the research and understand the insulin, they'll help you make it happen. With these great choices, parents don't need to ask their children to suffer more. It's a new century, thank goodness.

Meters 101

Other than insulin, perhaps the biggest breakthrough in treating diabetes in the twentieth century was the invention, improvement, and marketing of the blood glucose meter. Before meters, parents had little real clue to what even average blood sugars were. They went on lab draws that were weeks old or on urine tests that were marginal at best at pinpointing blood glucose levels. Meters changed it all, but it took time.

Building a Market

For years, engineers across the country and around the world had been dabbling with the concept of blood glucose meters. Finally, someone came up with the first model. However, few families had access to the technology, and those who did struggled with it. Blood was put directly on the meter (now there's an "eww factor" today's parents cannot fathom) and they were very expensive.

Although meters were introduced to the market in the 1970s, they did not come of age (i.e., become widely covered by health insurance) until after the results of the Diabetes Control and Complications Trial were released in 1993. This study conducted by the National Institute of Diabetes and Digestive and Kidney Diseases proved without much doubt that tighter control through better knowledge drastically cut the rate of complications in people with diabetes. It became clear at that time that better tools would not only be more humane for those suffering with diabetes, but they would also save the world hundreds of millions of dollars in costs associated with long-term care of people with diabetes.

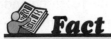 **Fact**

> The first blood glucose meter was the Ames Reflectance Meter, which hit the market in 1971, weighed two pounds, and took more than a minute to give a reading. Today, more than thirty brands of meters exist with some weighing mere ounces and taking five seconds for a reading.

More important, the study paved the way for meters to be covered by insurance, which unlocked the profit possibilities for technology companies. With that study's results, the race for the technology market share was on, and patients with diabetes were—and continue to be—the constant winners.

Today's Choices

Jumping ahead to the new century, meters now come in every shape, size, and pace. Deciding which one is right for you is personal and can really only be done through word of mouth and hands-on experience. It's possible to own a meter that counts down in five seconds. It is possible to own one that tucks into even the tiniest short-shorts pocket. Most meters have long memories and can store all kinds of patterns and information. Most have software so you can download readings and patterns to your computer and e-mail them to your medical team. It all comes down to personal preference. As always, ask your child which meter he likes and why. Take his opinions into account and consideration. But, the final choice should be yours. (See Chapter 18 for teens and pump manipulation issues.)

While some families use a variety of meters at one time, it's a good idea to stick to the same brand. Readings can vary a tiny bit from meter to meter, and most insurance will only cover one type of strip per month. If you decide to make a change, you may want to change out all the meters you have.

Which begs the question: What about using just one meter at all times? While this is generally a great idea, since it will keep all of your child's numbers in the same meter, it's not always possible. Ask yourself if you want your child carrying a meter to and from school, or would you rather she keeps one at home and one at school. Most parents opt for the latter, giving them one item less to forget on a school day morning.

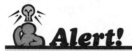

Alert!

For the most part, you should almost never have to pay for a meter. Most insurance plans cover one per year, and most medical teams have samples to give out. Meter companies make their profits on the strips, not the meters. Look for meter freebies at all times.

Glucagon 101

It's your worst fear. No parent wants to have to use a glucagon kit on their child, and chances are you'll never have to use it. However, being prepared for possibilities is what life with diabetes is all about, so understanding how, when, and why to use a glucagon kit is a must for all parents and caregivers of children with diabetes.

What Is It?

When the body's blood sugar goes low, it automatically secretes a hormone called glucagon. Glucagon helps the body rush glucose to where it is needed and fights off low blood sugar in emergency situations. This process happens naturally in people without diabetes. People with diabetes need to help their body make this happen in a severe low, and the glucagon kit is the tool to do that.

A glucagon kit holds a vial of liquid, a powdery substance that is actually one milligram of the hormone, and a needle. It also contains both written and pictorial instructions. Parents need to become familiar with their glucagon kit from the start.

When and How to Use It

Glucagon is used to ward off a seizure from dangerously low blood sugar levels. If your child is low and cannot ingest any kind of carbs, including juice or gels, it's time to pull out the kit. The dosing is prescribed, but it is not vital to stick to it. For the most part, children under forty pounds get half the vial, and anyone over forty pounds gets the entire vial.

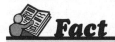 *Fact*

Many parents are frightened into thinking they must follow the dosing instructions precisely. Don't worry, you cannot overdose on glucagon, so in a pinch or a panic, just give the entire shot. You can always correct your child's high blood glucose level once the emergency is over.

Some doctors recommend older kids and adults take half the shot first and then the other half twenty minutes later if it is still needed as a way to reduce the rebound high that many experience after a low. Talk to your endocrinology team about what dose they'd rather you give your child, should an emergency arise. Write it down on the instructions inside the kit so it's there in an emergency.

When giving a child (or adult) glucagon, always place the person on her side. Glucagon can cause some vomiting. Give the shot in the arm or leg in a fatty tissue spot much like where you'd give an insulin injection.

If you're calm enough, wait out a call to 911. Most children and adults recover within fifteen minutes. But if you feel the panic and worry is too much, dial away. It's okay to need reassurance; she's your child, after all.

In the end, most parents who have given glucagon say even with the best preparation, they were frightened in the moment. Don't be afraid to ask for help if you feel you need it.

Where to Keep Glucagon Kits

While parents would love to scatter the earth with glucagon kits, you have to have a realistic plan. One should always be in your home in an easy-to-access spot that everyone knows. Another should be at school, in a place that is easy to get to for the person who will administer it. You may want one more to send with your child on activities such as sleepovers and parties and play dates. Even if you cannot train a friend to use it, you can have it there for emergency personnel to have access to should the need arise. Follow the old adage: The only place you'll need a glucagon kit is where you don't have it. Always have one within reach.

New Devices: Today and on the Horizon

Never before has the landscape been richer for new devices to help families deal with diabetes. Technological and pharmaceutical companies have gotten a taste of the market, and that's good news for parents and families. While some products are still in the conceptual stage, others are being tested or even on the market. A cure is the goal, but better treatment will help along the way.

Continuous Meters

For the most part, continuous meters track interstitial glucose, giving a blood sugar reading about every five seconds, and a visible display of what the reading is and if the blood glucose is trending up or down. Those who have used them say it's changed the way they treat their diabetes.

Right now, a continuous meter means a second infusion site and a second device either worn on the body or carried with the person.

Industry is hoping to make the meter part of pumps in the future. In all likelihood, in a few years these continuous meters will become the standard of care, once patients and providers learn how to use the data they provide. Clinical trials in children with Type 1 diabetes are under way throughout the United States. Ask your endocrinologist for details. ⬦

Ketone-Reading Meters

Until a few years ago, ketones could only be read in the urine, a practice that's vague and not timely (urine ketones are about two hours behind what is going on in the bloodstream). Today, the ketone meter means an instant reading of exactly what the ketone level is in your bloodstream. Medical teams love families that use these meters since in high blood sugar situations, this up-to-the-minute information can assist the teams to help the families keep kids out of the ER.

Right now the only ketone meter on the market is by Abbott, and the strips are expensive. If you can, get insurance to cover about thirty a month and always refill them each month even if you don't use them. In that way, you'll have enough on hand if a ketone emergency comes along. Again, most endocrinology teams have meters to give you, which means that you'll only need to buy the strips, perhaps with an insurance copay.

Continuous Glucose Monitors

A CGM is, quite simply, a sensor that is placed below the skin and attached to a transmitter that continually checks blood sugars and transmits them to a receptor, either part of an insulin pump or a separate device carried along or held. Because the sensor is checking constantly, the person with diabetes can see on a screen, not only a current reading of what their blood sugar is, but a graph showing how her blood sugars are trending over the day. At press time, CGMs were quite new but being used by adults and children with diabetes with great success.

Using a CGM, parents of diabetic children can know how their child trends through the day and therefore make smart adjustments to insulin. Having a place where the parents can see, on a screen, which foods make their child spike and how far, can help parents make diet decisions or up insulin doses for certain foods. A device that constantly checks (and is reliable) can also help parents give their child more freedom.

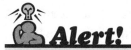

Alert!

Right now, the CGM devices are not covered by insurance and most families using them are paying out of pocket about $200 a month. However, some individuals have fought with insurance companies and have been able to win coverage, and groups like the JDRF are working toward making coverage a law.

For most, the notion of another device can be worrisome, but some children find, particularly in the case of the Medtronic Min-iMed System, that it's not as overbearing as one might think. In the case of the MiniMed, a sensor the size of a pump site goes in and is connected to a transmitter about the size of two-thirds of a playing card and about an eighth of an inch think. This transmitter is taped down to the body and is barely visible under clothing. Because the readings come through on the actual MiniMed pump, there is no additional device to wear or carry. Just push a button on your pump and you see your reading. MiniMed expects to debut a smaller trans-mitter some time in early 2007.

In the case of the DexCom, a similar site is put in, and a smaller transmitter is attached, about the size of two fingers. That transmits to a second piece, an oval-shaped device about the size of a pump, which can be carried in your pocket or purse but must stay within five feet of your body.

The Freestyle Navigator is similar to the DexCom in its working, and also requires an added piece to be carried. It is in clinical stud-ies now.

Like pumps, choosing a CGM is a personal choice. If you are interested, let your child see all the models and consider how each would impact his life. In the end, let him help you make the decision. It's his body, after all.

Challenges of CMG

For now, those trying this new technology are finding it amazing and yet challenging. Having two sites in a child at all times is tricky: You'll need to work hard at rotating so as not to build up scar tissue. And learning to use the CGM as a tool and not a device that you become a slave to is important too. But, most who have tried it have found it to be life changing.

Some children, however, find that a CGM is too much. They don't want a second site and they don't want to have to know their blood sugars all the time. Another challenge is that, while most would like to think so, a CGM does not totally eliminate finger pricks, as they are needed for calibration. But, used well, a CGM can mean only two finger pricks a day on an average day (keeping in mind that, when in doubt, a back up finger prick is always advised). In the end, as always, your child's personal well being should come first.

What They Can Mean

If the theory that regulated blood sugars equate to an offset of complications is true, CGMs could mean even less chance of kidney failure and other such complications. They can also mean a better grasp on what diabetes does to the body on a daily basis. No one is certain of what happens between blood sugar readings, but now, those who choose to use a CGM will have that knowledge. However this knowledge also brings the challenge for parents and patients not to overreact to readings and to look at trends instead.

It is the hope of scientists that someday, the CGM and the pump will work as a team, reading blood sugars and then giving insulin as needed without the patient doing anything but wearing them. This is in the future, but being worked on.

CHAPTER 7

All about Pumps

T hey are the biggest news in daily pediatric diabetes care in the past ten years, and one of the most important decisions you'll make as you and your child work toward finding the best way to deal with diabetes on a daily basis. They are insulin pumps or continuous subcutaneous insulin infusion (CSII), as they are called clinically. Pumps have changed everything for kids and diabetes, and at least considering one for your child at any age is a must.

What Is an Insulin Pump?

An insulin pump is a pager-like device that delivers fast-acting insulin to the body through a cannula and tubing in two ways; a preprogrammed basal rate that delivers small amounts continuously over a twenty-four-hour period, and a bolus that the wearer or the parent or caregiver of the wearer pushes buttons to deliver at needed times such as meals and when high blood sugar levels occur.

The site or infusion area, which includes the cannula and tubing is inserted either by hand or with an insertion tool and is changed about every three days. Most children say the insertion hurts no more than an insulin shot. The pump can be disconnected from the site at any time and reconnected with an easy click. Insulin travels from the pump through the tubing and into the body.

A pump is not a cure for diabetes, and while it does replace shots, it does not replace finger pricks for blood

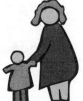

glucose readings. In other words, while pumps are a great delivery system for insulin, they do not regulate blood sugars on their own, a common misconception by the general public.

Pump Freedom

A pump does, however, allow the user to have a freer schedule. Since there is fast-acting insulin in the pump, there are no peak times; in other words, there are no times when eating or snacking is a must. Since a person with a pump only needs to do a math equation and push some buttons when he wants to eat, a pump means you can eat or—to the surprise of people with diabetes who have been living on shots for years—you can *not eat* whenever you'd like. Pumping is by no means complete freedom. It comes with its own set of demands that, while different from shots, can be demanding as well.

How Pumps Came to Market

Pumps were first made available to the public around 1980, but only adults could wear them and users of the large, bulky pumps were few and far between. In 1985, MiniMed introduced the 507, the first sleeker, more modern pump that would be the catalyst for many people with diabetes to turn to pumps instead of shots. Still, parents who wanted pumps on their children were few and far between, and they had to either work hard to find an endocrine team willing to help them out or pretty much do it on their own.

Even once the child barrier was broken, most pediatric endocrinology teams held to a belief that "when you can drive a car, you can drive a pump." It wasn't until parents began truly pushing in the late 1990s that more and more kids started pumping. Even then, many parents had to work hard to convince their medical teams to let them give it a try.

Pump companies helped families out, too, for obvious reasons. The pediatric market would be a boon for them. This push actually, for a short time, caused medical teams to hold back, not trusting the motives of the companies. In addition, until recently, there was no data that pumps were safe and effective in young children. This lack of efficacy data slowed adoption of pumps in children. Eventually, large studies were published that showed how pumps could be effectively used in children. As a result, pediatric endocrinology teams began to put more patients on pumps.

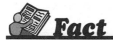 **Fact**

One of the first known young children on a pump was a three-year-old girl in upstate New York in 1985. It would be decades before having children on pumps became the norm in diabetes care.

Still, parents kept pushing until they made it happen for their children. Naturally, the more successes medical teams saw, the more willing they were to come on board. Today, pumps are available to kids of all ages.

The Pros and Cons of Pumping

So, is pumping right for your child? To know the answer, you have to consider the good, the not-so-good, and the challenging aspects of pumping.

The Great Things about Pumps

The best thing about pumping, most families will tell you, is the freedom. For any child tied to a meal plan and shot schedule, the idea of complete freedom when it comes to scheduling life is a dream come true. Children are often freer to take part in other activities, too. Although a friend's parent probably would not want to give your child a shot, pushing a button on a pump would be something she could handle. Picture yourself sending little Bobby over to a friend's house for lunch. If he were on shots, you might have to send along a pre-drawn needle for the other parent to help administer. With the pump, you can simply tell the parent what number to push on the pump, or better yet, call Bobby and talk him through it as the other parent supervises. Many parents find the pump helps ease their worries when it comes to playtime.

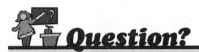

Question?

Will a pump conspicuously show my child's diabetes to the world?
Not necessarily. Pumps can slide easily into pockets, and there are a multitude of clip-on cases available to hold them. Most kids don't mind showing them, but if they want to be discreet, it's easy to do.

Another pro to pumping, for parents, is the ability to tweak insulin doses and carbohydrate ratios to a degree that simply can't be done with shots. With a pump, you can adjust doses up and down by .05 units. Imagine trying to draw up to that tiny amount on a syringe. It's nearly impossible. With basal adjustments, you can change your child's insulin input every half hour if necessary. Best yet, when your child runs high, you can bring her down at the push of a button rather than having to worry about what other insulin type might be peaking in upcoming hours. Done well, pumping almost always means a decrease in A1c results, and it often means getting that lower number while allowing a child more freedom.

Pumps can mean fewer lows (hypoglycemia), too. One of the big concerns that pediatric endocrinologists had in the early years was that pumps would cause lows; however, it has been documented that kids on pumps tend to have fewer lows than kids on shots.

The Things That Make You Worry

Pumps are not all parties and freedom. Pumping means your child is only on fast-acting insulin. In other words, should the pump fail, the site clog, or something else go wrong, your child has no "safety net" insulin to fall back on in the absence of the short-acting insulin. This can be frightening to some parents, but the reality is, if you check your child's blood sugars regularly (at least every four hours during the day, and at night from time to time), you're not going to let your child go too far into a dangerous high blood sugar situation.

In addition, a child could develop ketones faster than she did on shots. The long-acting insulin is not there to back things up, so ketones can come on quickly.

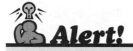

Alert!

Always correct a high blood sugar with ketones with a shot. Never depend on the pump and the site in a ketone situation. The shot is sure to work, and you'll be able to check on the pump and site in the meantime.

That means that kids on pumps absolutely have to check their blood sugars regularly. If you're a parent who is fine with, say, three blood checks a day and don't want to add more, the pump is not the right choice for you and your child.

Another worry can be the notion of change. Often, children who have had diabetes for years are hesitant to make a treatment change and would rather stick to their tried-and-true shots. While it's a good idea to encourage children to try change, you cannot force a child to do so.

Parents might also worry about the pump if their child is active in sports. The good news is that while some sports, such as football, might require a child to unhook during play, there is no sport that rules out using a pump, since you can detach it for as much as an entire day if done properly (how to do so is discussed later in the chapter). For some kids and parents, however, the stress of disconnecting is too much, and they opt not to pump.

Lipohypertrophy

Lipohypertrophy is the bulging of an area of the skin due to the scar tissue and fat accumulation that forms when a person injects himself or inserts a pump site in the same spot over and over again. Kids can tend toward this habit for a number of reasons. Perhaps they don't like to try new spots, and a spot used over and over can lose its feeling (don't let anyone fool you; diabetes *can* hurt).

The danger is that insulin has a harder time being absorbed in these damaged areas. Your child must rotate spots, and you as parent must watch him and make sure he does. Ideally, insulin should go into fresh sites as often as possible. This alone might contribute to a decrease in your child's A1c.

Don't Fret at Saying No to Pumping

The community advocating pumps for children is a vocal and passionate one. As more and more children pump, you'll hear more and more about it for your child. If you do decide it's not for you, don't let anyone tell you the decision is wrong. As always, the person who knows what is best for your child and your family is you. Trust your gut and go with it.

Ages and Pump Issues

While it has taken decades to get to this point, pumps are now an acceptable therapy for children of all ages: toddlers, teens, and even, in some case, infants. Each age group has its own set of challenges that parents and caregivers need to address when it comes to pumping, but each age also has its benefits.

Tiny Tots

Although toddlers and babies were the last to receive professional approval for pumping, they could possibly benefit the most from the therapy. First, they are almost always in the direct care and supervision of a parent or another caring adult. This means the child will always be within arm's reach of an adult who knows how to work the pump.

Toddlers and babies, too, can be difficult (at best) to convince to conform to a meal plan. A pump gives them the freedom to nurse or eat or nibble the same as any tiny tot would.

A pump, too, can mean that parents can give their child tiny, tiny doses with incredible accuracy. That's a big win with little ones.

What about wearing the pump? Most pumps come with a lock-out option so that toddlers cannot push the buttons and make anything happen. There are also holsters available so kids can wear them on their backs where they cannot reach or see them.

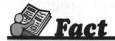 **Fact**

For great choices in pump-carrying products, go to *www.uniaccs .com*. This company specializes in making products to help people carry their pumps comfortably, privately, and in a way that fits their lifestyles. Oftentimes, all a child needs is a cute way to hold their pump to make them happy with it.

A toddler in day care will need a caring provider who is willing to learn all about the pump and how to help her get through the day on the pump. Include the care provider in the training your pump company will give you when you purchase it. You'll also want to keep her in the loop on the pump and any changes that come along.

Elementary School Children

The elementary years can be tricky years for pumping, but most parents find it's worth the effort to make it work out. The plain truth is your child will have to check blood sugars more often on a pump. If your school insists that a child must be in the nurse's office to do that, he may have to leave the classroom more frequently. As discussed in Chapter 10, you can find ways to make that work, including getting an aide who is trained in diabetes and pumps placed in your child's classroom.

Bolusing (another name for a dose of insulin used to cover meals or lower blood sugars) and correcting can be tricky for children this age as well. Make sure you keep your school nurse or aide up to speed on any bolus rate and carb ratio changes you make over the school year.

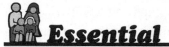 **Essential**

> Colored stickers work well for pumping kids who bring lunch. Write each food item's carb total on a sticker and place it on the wrapping. Ask your child to keep the stickers from the foods she eats during the day and then add them up to do the meal bolus.

Some parents let a child do boluses at an early age. It's a good idea to at least have someone—the nurse, a teacher, or an aide—check on your child's math and the bolus. It can be confusing.

The good news about kids this age is they generally think pumps are just plain cool. It's usually easy to convince this age group to try one out, and they are, for the most part, open with their schoolmates about wearing one. Often, boys and girls see older teens with pumps at diabetes camp and, wanting to be like the cool older kids, come home asking for one.

Teens

Teens who have had diabetes for years or who were newly diagnosed can be tougher to convince. They are less likely to be willing to have something so seemingly obvious on their bodies and may balk initially at the idea. If you can, get your teen to talk to other teens who pump. Have the other teens show your son or daughter how the pump can be worn comfortably and discreetly. Have them talk about how much easier it is to be a teen with the freedom of a pump.

You can also show your teen a list of famous cool people who wear pumps. Pro ballplayers, former Miss Americas, and many others celebrities wear pumps, and that might help them consider the possibility.

Also remind your teen: It cannot hurt to try. If they hook up and decide weeks later they prefer shots, they can go back to shots. It's their choice in the end.

Where to Begin

Once you've made the decision to have your child try pumping, the process can be intimidating. Your medical team and pump company are both ready to walk you through the entire process. You can make it happen smoothly.

Choosing a Pump

Parents worry about this aspect of beginning pumping almost more than any other part. The irony is there really is no need for stress. Pumps are like automobiles: They all work pretty well and pretty much the same. It's up to your child and you, based on the style and options you like, to choose a pump.

Don't agonize too much about what's on the horizon in pump options either. There is always going to be a new model down the line, and there will never (at this point anyway) be a time that the best model for all time is here. Choose one you and your child like, and get going.

Start-up Time

You'll need to set a start-up date with your medical team and look to make that happen. Some teams are booked solid getting kids going on pumps, and it may be a little time before your team can schedule you. Don't be disappointed if you have to wait. You can use that time to read up and learn all you can on pumping.

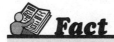 **Fact**

The bible of pump therapy is *Pumping Insulin* by John Walsh. If you're considering or beginning pumping, you should have this book on your bookshelf.

Expect your Certified Diabetes Educator to be your main point person on the start-up. Your endocrinologist will be in on things as well, but usually the CDE is in charge.

Is it better to start at a certain time of year? Some families prefer to do it in the summer, when they have their child with them at all times. Others like the school year because of the set schedule. It's a personal decision, and one you should think through. It's not a good idea to start pumping just days before you're heading away on vacation. Nor is it a good idea to start during a time in your lives that is disrupted for other reasons, such as a recent divorce or another illness in the family. Make sure you can clear your schedule for what some like to call "pumpternity leave." This time will be like having a new baby; only it will just be a few days before you have that baby sleeping through the night.

Your medical team will most likely ask you to check your child every couple of hours all night long for the first few nights to get a feel for any adjustments that need to be made in the basal rates or in the bolus ratio. The team will help you look at all the numbers and information and get things just right. It will happen, just give it time.

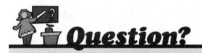 **Question?**

Do I need to take time off work to help my child with a pump start-up?
It's not essential, but it's a good idea to take a few days off for this. The start-up appointment will take almost a full day, and you'll also be up nights for at least a few days. This disruption in daily life is often more than some people want to deal with after working all day long, and so they take days off to deal with the start-up.

Many parents report a certain familiar stress at new pump time. The changes, learning curve, and panic can bring them back to original diagnosis time. But don't fret, this should—and will, in most cases—pass quickly. When you see your child thrive on this new technology, you'll realize this was not a trauma like the diagnosis but rather a giant leap forward.

Cool Pump Tricks for Everyone

Pumpers have figured out a lot of things over the years and are always more than willing to share them. Finding those hints and trying them out is all part of making the pump work for your child.

Where to Find Tricks

There's a wealth of information out there, starting first, as always, with your support groups and friends with children with diabetes. Ask them to share their tricks with you, such as where to put a pump, how to figure out the detaching puzzle, and where to hide a pump on a body.

Talk to your CDE, too, about the basics as well as the tricks he's learned from other patients. In time, you'll have your own tips and tricks to share.

Try These at Home

Girls find that sports bras are the golden ticket to wearing a pump with some clothing. The pump can be tucked into the middle back of the bra comfortably, where it won't slip and won't show. Some small girls have even started wearing sports bras early, just to hold pumps in place.

Families who vacation far away often find that by calling the pump company ahead of time, they'll gladly send a backup loaner pump. That way, if your child's pump fails in a distant place, you'll have a spare on hand to keep things going.

Kids who like to disconnect for sports find that by checking every two hours, they can go almost all day without their pump on. If their levels are a bit high at checking time, they simply need to click the pump on, put a correction bolus through, and then take it off again. But they must check every two hours to make this work.

Some kids like to use a variety of site choices for different needs. You can order as many different types as you want at refill time. Consider ordering a few types and letting your child vary which he uses.

Saying No to Pumping

Pump parents and patients are like revivalists: They believe they've found the Holy Grail. But like anything else in diabetes, pumping is a personal decision and in the end, it is up to you and your child to decide if it is right for you.

Why Not?

Some children and parents or caregivers prefer the routine of shots and even meal plans. While some may say you're crazy, the fact is, what works for you is what works for you. Most doctors agree that the perfect way to use a pump is with a schedule and meal plan, yet for the most part, pumpers do not follow this advice. That's because most are after the freedom, and there's nothing wrong with that. But if you like to stick to a plan and feel your child does not want change, you can just say no.

Some children just don't want something attached to their bodies. Also, some kids have been in the routine of shots for so long, they fear change. In the end, there's no forcing this issue.

How to Say No

It won't be easy. The passion of pumpers is almost unimaginable. You may have to listen to as many silly comments from them as you've had to from people who don't know about diabetes. But if you explain that you have indeed researched it and it is not for you, any polite person should back off.

One thing not to accept is a no if you want a yes. If your medical team says you cannot put your child on a pump, demand an answer that you understand, and then search for a new team that will help you out. Pumping is personal, but today with what the world knows about kids and pumps, it should be available to everyone.

CHAPTER 8

The First Weeks

Y ou did it. You walked out of that hospital and back into the world you knew BD (before diabetes). Yet somehow, everything seems different. You perceive land mines everywhere: in food stores, in restaurants, at the playground, in your own kitchen, and yes, in your bedrooms. You take baby steps, figuring out how to dose insulin, read blood sugars, manage meals, and just plain live with diabetes. The first weeks at home with diabetes are a moment-by-moment learning experience; one that, done right, can lay a foundation for smoother times to follow.

Settling In

The first days at home are a whirlwind. Friends all want to stop by; everyone wants to help out. You just want to figure out how you're going to keep your child not just healthy but alive. Parents or caregivers have different reactions at the start. Some feel empowered and happy to have figured out what was wrong with their child. For them, the first days are often a relief, and tougher times may follow. Others, more commonly, are frightened, worried, and overwhelmed with the life adjustments they are about to make and the added responsibility they now have.

In either case, it's a good idea to ask friends to give you and your child some breathing space. The key to raising a child with diabetes successfully is finding a new normal, a new way to add all this to his life in a way

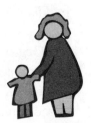

that feels somewhat like any other life. That's no small task. Telling friends you appreciate their compassion but you need some space is a wise choice at this point. If they must help, ask them to take one of your other children for a play date, or go out and find a good diabetes book for you. You'll need this time to settle in and adjust to your new role as parent and medical caretaker.

 ## Essential

A good way to bring your friends into the loop is to have a "Getting to know diabetes" get-together. Invite all your good friends and parents of your child's good friends and give them a short course in diabetes 101 and what it will mean for your child's play dates at their house. This will cut down on the number of times you have to explain.

You may also want to ask a relative or close friend to screen calls and e-mail for you for the first week. Explaining yourself repeatedly can be exhausting. You'll need all your strength to get things in place at home, and a message from a family member or friend to concerned folks will be enough for now.

Organizing, Storing, and Toting the Supplies

Looking at all of the tools of the trade of diabetes can shock a parent. You can easily fill two large kitchen drawers with the supplies and tools you now need to keep your child healthy. Finding a smart way to organize and tote them around is a great first step toward integrating diabetes into your life as seamlessly as possible.

Organization

It's time to scope out a place for diabetes central. This will be the place in your home where the bulk of diabetes supplies are stored. Some parents opt for a kitchen cabinet, others for a couple of kitchen drawers. Utility closet shelves or a cabinet in a laundry room or powder room are also good choices. Whatever space you select, clean it out, empty it, and make sure it is only for diabetes supplies.

Drawers work well because it's easy to locate what you are looking for. Cabinets, however, have more space and hold more. If small children are involved, you will need to consider childproofing the space immediately. Syringes, lancets, and other supplies are not something you ever want a child toying with.

Once you've cleaned your space, fill it with your supplies in categories. Test strips and meter supplies such as lancets, control solution, and backup meters should be stored in one area. In another area, place syringes, alcohol swabs, and other site-preparation solutions or wipes. At the very front of your space, place your glucagon and backup glucagons, as well as a package of glucose tablets or another fast-acting sugar, such as Skittles or jelly beans. Just under those supplies, place a reminder sheet that spells out what to do in case of a low blood sugar emergency.

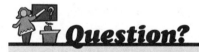 *Question?*

How do I get more than a few of everything?
In most cases, your insurance will cover everything your endocrinology team writes a script for. Talk to your team about the amount of things you'd like to have, add a bit to pad that amount, and ask for a script for that.

In a third area in the same storage space, place ketone-testing supplies, such as ketone strips, a ketone meter, and ketone meter strips. Always keep a set of the instructions to translate the ketone results in that same place. It's amazing what can flee your mind when you are in a panic.

Now you need to turn to other parts of your home and life. It's a good idea to assume you'll be running out in a rush from time to time.

For that reason, pack a diabetes travel kit and keep it packed and ready at all times. It should hold a few syringes, some lancets, alcohol prep wipes, glucose tablets, and a glucagon kit. Back that up by placing yet another glucagon and syringe in the glove compartment of your car. Also, place ketone strip bottles in the medicine cabinet of each bathroom, and glucose tablets in a drawer in your child's bedroom. This way, you'll have everything close to you at all times and seldom will you forget. (Although, forget you will. We are all human.)

Storage

Most diabetes supplies will stay well in a cool, dark place. Things like meter strips and glucagon do not need to be kept chilled, and as long as they are protected from direct sun and high temperatures, they'll be fine in almost any spot.

Insulin, on the other hand, needs to be handled carefully. Insulin that gets too hot or too cold can be unusable, and the only way you'll find out is when your child's blood sugar goes high despite having been given a dose.

It's best to store insulin in your refrigerator. Most folks choose the butter dish area. Ask a person with diabetes to try to find the insulin in your house, and the first place she'll look is in that butter dish. That is because that area gives you the cold of the fridge in a kinder, gentler (keep that butter softer) kind of way. It's easy to find there, too. It peeks out at you at eye level and never gets pushed behind the juice boxes or milk cartons or leftover Chinese food.

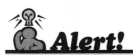

Alert!

It is not a wise choice to store extra insulin in your car or purse. Cars and purses that are left in cars can heat up quickly. You'll have to be diligent about remembering always to bring insulin along when you head out of the house. Remember, the only time you'll need emergency insulin is when you don't have it.

Insulin does not need to be kept cold. In fact, when it comes to pumps, many endocrinology teams recommend patients use room-temperature insulin. The rule is that once opened, insulin stays good up to three months when refrigerated. At room temperature, it stays good for only one month. Sealed insulin, refrigerated, is good up to the expiration date on the bottle. Sealed at room temperature, it stays good for only one month. Most parents of newly diagnosed children or of very small children opt to keep insulin in the fridge at all times, since they use such a small amount.

If you do keep your insulin at room temperature, make sure you store it in a cool, dry, dark place. Direct sunlight or exposure to any kind of heat or cold could dilute the insulin. Tucked to the side in a spice cabinet, or on a shelf in a medicine cabinet is a good bet.

Keep in mind, though, that some children complain that cold insulin hurts more during injections. If this is the case with your child, keep one vial out and dispose of it at month's end, even if it is not completely empty.

Totes

So what about carrying all those supplies around? Parents and caregivers new to diabetes can look down at what's needed to take along with you and feel like only a Sherpa could do the job. With good planning and good equipment, you'll find that bringing it all along is possible.

First, shop for some small carrying cases. There are cases specifically for diabetes supplies that you can find at your pharmacy or online. These cases are handy because they have special loops just the size of your insulin bottles and compartments for each item needed. They are helpful in that each compartment reminds you of something you need to have.

You will always need to carry a meter. New meters are small and portable; some even slip into a child's jeans pocket. But it's a good idea to encourage your child, and yourself, to carry them in their case. Some girls like to find cute wristlets that are popular now to carry their meter and glucose tabs in. Boys seem to prefer large pocketed shorts or jeans to tuck their meter case into.

When you are with your child, you should always bring along insulin, syringes, a glucagon kit, a meter, and extra strips. Meter batteries are a good idea to tuck away in your purse or glove compartment. You never know when you're going to need them.

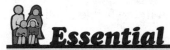

Essential

Caboodle cases, those bright plastic cases girls love to carry makeup or craft supplies in, are a dream case for diabetes supplies. The many-sized cubbies are just right for all the supplies, and kids feel good about toting them along to parties or sleepovers.

What should you expect your child to tote along when he's out playing? The rule is simple: If he's in the neighborhood, he only needs to have a fast-acting glucose supply on hand, and perhaps (if it's not too bothersome) his meter.

Outside the neighborhood, your child must understand that she needs all her supplies within close distance. This can be a bone of contention, particularly for children struggling with this new part of their identity. Work with your child to come up with a plan. If she carries a cell phone and you will be close, perhaps she can just carry a meter, strips, and glucose. If the readings were high, she could call you to come meet her with insulin and a syringe. If she is playing in another neighborhood, perhaps a good friend would be willing to let you temporarily keep supplies at her house while your child is playing.

Storage and toting of supplies to and from school will be discussed in Chapter 10.

How to Use Your Medical Team During the First Weeks

The hardest part about leaving the hospital and heading home is cutting the direct cord with that medical team you met and worked with in the hospital. It can be frightening for parents to head out on their own. It's important to remember that the team might not live in your house, but they are (or should be) available to help you at any hour, not just through these crucial first weeks, but for all the time they treat your child. A good pediatric endocrinology team has someone on call 24/7 to help you, and they never question your need for help.

When to Call

Your team will most likely send you home from the hospital visit with specific orders, target range glucose levels, and guidelines on when and why to call them. Target ranges vary with the child and with age. In the beginning, medical teams aim a little higher than average for blood glucose levels to keep your child safe as you learn to give insulin and monitor blood sugar.

The insulin doses you are sent home with could change within days. In the past, children were always sent home on a mix of long-acting insulin called NPH and short-acting insulin called regular. When fast-acting insulin, such as Humalog and Novolog, was approved for children in 1998, and when the nonpeaking Lantus was introduced circa 2001, doctors had more options for newly diagnosed kids. (Insulin choices and their uses are discussed in Chapter 6.) Whatever combination your child's doctor sends him home on, expect to make changes in dose amounts as the days go on.

Your team will ask you to keep a detailed logbook of your child's blood sugars, what she eats, and what activities she takes part in. These notes will be crucial in the first weeks and in the long run as well.

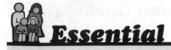 **Essential**

> An easy way to make your logbook simpler to read is to use a four-color pen, available at most stores. Write low numbers in red, high numbers in blue, within-target numbers in green, and all notes in black. Instead of having to study numbers for patterns or trends, the colors will make them jump off the page for you.

You can expect to talk to your child's endocrinologist or Certified Diabetes Educator at least once in the first week, but don't be afraid to call more often. Most parents panic the first time their child is high or low, and doctors expect that call. The call will be worthwhile for you, even if it's just for reassurance.

Have Your Information at Hand

Once the first times pass, it's a good idea to look for patterns before calling your team for advice. See a relatively high number after lunch one day? Feed your child about the same meal the next day and see if it happens again. If it does, a change in insulin dose may be needed, and you'll need advice to make that decision. Seeing a lot of lows? Then it's time to call again. Your child may be getting more active or going into a honeymoon period and you'll need to cut back on an insulin dose.

Any time your child has an unexplained low or high in the middle of the night, it's a good idea to call. Any time your child tests positive for ketones, you should call your medical team right away.

Planning a first family trip? That's another good time to call your team, although nonemergency calls should be limited to regular hours, and not go to on-call doctors during off hours. The same goes for prescription refill requests. Unless you drop all your insulin on the floor and need it immediately, plan to make those benign calls during working hours. Your team will thank you for it.

What if you're just feeling overwhelmed or worried? Call them. Learning to care for a child with diabetes can be stressful, and you'll need all the professional help you can get. One day, as time ticks by, you'll find you don't need to call all the time anymore. Until then, use your resources as you see fit.

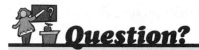

Question?

What if my team does not answer?
If you do not have a team with at least one member available at any hour of any day, you may want to consider changing practices. Diabetes knows no business hours, and you cannot risk your child's health because her medical help isn't available.

That First High Blood Sugar

It's going to happen—and you're going to panic. As much as you'd like to keep your child's blood sugar in the allotted target range, it's just too difficult to do 100 percent of the time. So the day comes; you prick your child's finger and squeeze the drop, wait for the count-down expecting to see, say, 104 (isn't that what the meters always say on the commercials?) and instead up pops 342. What's a parent to do?

First, as difficult as it may sound, don't panic. A high blood sugar is a time to respond immediately, but it is not an immediate crisis. Even if you don't say it out loud and you panic inside, your child will most likely sense that. Try to brace yourself ahead of time for the times you see those high numbers. When it is above acceptable range, take action.

Your medical team will tell you that if your child's level goes over a certain number—most choose 260 or higher—you should always check for ketones. If your child is above that chosen range, check for ketones immediately. If you do call your medical team, the first thing they will ask is if you checked. A high blood sugar reading is no good without ketone information. Once you know that, get out your logbook and study the day. Did your child eat something she has not eaten since diagnosis? Many children react differently to different foods (for instance, some kids go high a few hours after eating pasta or pizza). If your child has ketones, you must call your team right away. If your child does not have ketones and you feel confident that you know what caused the high and what the correction ration of insulin should be, you can make a correction and check the blood sugar again in two hours.

 Essential

When reacting to a high blood sugar reading, always check your child's hands and make sure they were clean. More than a few parents and caregivers have panicked over what was actually some sugar or sweetener on a child's hand. When in doubt, wash up and check again.

Highs Happen

It is important for you and your child to realize that highs happen. There is a saying in the diabetes world: There is no such thing as a *bad* blood sugar. That's because any blood glucose reading is information that you can use to take action. Children need to understand early that diabetes is a relentless disease; even when they do their best, it will sometimes trip them up. Calling blood sugars good or bad can lead a child to think he did something wrong, or right, with his diabetes. You may want to let friends, family, and teachers know that they should never refer to a blood glucose reading as good or bad.

Children quickly become knowledgeable about their bodies and their blood glucose. Many children can feel their highs coming on. They feel hyperactive and thirsty, and they need to urinate frequently. Don't go on these feelings alone, however. More than one child has confused the feeling of a high blood sugar with a low. Use your meter.

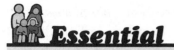

Essential

Never call a blood sugar good or bad. Readings are information only, not a judgment. Use the terms *high* or *low* instead, and your child will never feel judged. Insist others do this as well.

That First Low Blood Sugar

It is perhaps the thing parents new to the diabetes world fear the most: a low blood sugar. Severe low blood sugars are an immediate crisis because they can cause seizures and even death. The first time you see that meter read below 80 or even below 50, it can paralyze you with fear. Again, the key is to stay calm. You need to get fast-acting glucose into your child as quickly as possible. In the beginning, don't worry about overdoing it: A little bit of a high after a low is not uncommon. Choose an easy-to-digest fast-acting sugar.

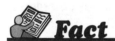

Fact

Good choices for fast-acting glucose include glucose tablets (available at most pharmacies), juice boxes, Skittles, and honey packets. Avoid chocolate; the fat slows the absorption process.

Treat your child with at least 15 grams of the carbohydrate you choose, and check her again in fifteen minutes. If she is still below normal, treat her again and check in another fifteen minutes. If you continue to have trouble bringing her up, call your medical team. Some people call this plan the "15–15 fix," an easy concept when you're learning to help care for your child.

Lows just before an activity like gym class or a sporting event usually mean you need to double your correction. Lows during the night are particularly important to treat with care. Some parents swear by giving a glass of whole milk along with a correction carbohydrate at night. The slow-releasing carbs and fat in the milk can help keep a child's blood sugar up until morning.

When It's a Crisis

What if your child's level gets so low he cannot ingest food or drink or respond to you? It's time to pull out the glucagon kit. Parents who have had to use it report that, at the time, it can be confusing and frightening. Ask your team if they have a spare expired glucagon you can practice on. At the very least, read through the instructions inside the case. They are in print and also, for panic moments, in picture form. Try to become familiar with the instructions and know that most parents never, ever have to use one.

If you do have to use glucagon and are alone and afraid, do not hesitate to call your medical team's emergency line as you work; you can also call 911 if you are truly afraid. Most low blood sugar emergencies, once treated with glucagon, are corrected within a few minutes, and the child does not need transportation or hospitalization. If you're brave enough, see it through. But if you call for emergency help, you are among the majority.

Nighttime Checks: How Many and How Often?

Nighttime checks are controversial in the diabetes parent's world. Some parents argue that you need to check at least once and many times more than once per night. Others say that nighttime checks are only necessary when it's been an unusual day or you are changing doses. As the weeks and months go by, you will decide what you are comfortable with, and how often you need to check at night.

In the beginning, let your medical team lead you on how often to check. Know though, that most parents do check at least once in the middle of the night in the first weeks. Being able to sleep through the night and let your child do so as well comes with experience and confidence.

Many children are lucky enough to feel their lows. Some children report having dreams of someone telling them they are low and that waking them up. But in the beginning, as you're getting used to trusting your instincts and knowing that your child will be fine for a night, you may want to check frequently.

How to Pull It Off

If you have a deft touch, your child need never wake up for a check. Many meters now have nighttime lights that illuminate the strip area, allowing you to see it in the dark. If you don't have one of those meters, put a night-light in your child's room near his bed. Finger-prick lancets are thin enough now that most children can sleep through them. Of course, if they are low, you get to experience the fun of forcing a child to eat in the middle of the night.

Some children insist on waking up and checking themselves. If this is the case, don't worry about it disrupting your child's sleep. Most children do not even recall the next morning that they even checked.

Can You Go Too Far?

There is such a thing as too much information, and too much intervention. Some caregivers report checking their child's blood sugar as many as fourteen times a day and three to four times a night. While it would be nice to be able to know all that information, it is important to remember that you—and your child—need to live a happy, normal life within the constraints of living with diabetes. Such activity on an extended basis could be a sign of psychological trouble. If you find yourself needing to check this often, you should discuss it with your medical team and your social worker.

It is acceptable to check that often when your child is ill, particularly with a stomach bug (see Chapter 19 for sick day details), or if she is beginning a new activity, such as skiing or hiking a long distance. It is also wise to check more than once during a night if your child had a severe low that day.

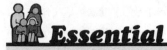

Essential

Checking can be fun! Set up a bingo card with all kinds of numbers you might see on the meter (high, low, and in range). Every time your child does a check, mark the number down. Give him a prize when he gets bingo!

The first weeks can be dicey, and with everything being so new, even a trip to the supermarket can bring stress and tears. Taking it one step and one challenge at a time will help you make it to the next step: gaining confidence in your skills as a parent of a child with diabetes. Remember when you brought home a newborn. At first, everything scared you and you could barely sleep through the night. But as days go by and your skills and education grew, so did your confidence. Eventually, you all slept through the night.

CHAPTER 9

Family Dynamics

T he impact of the diabetes diagnosis is not limited to the child with the disease. From siblings struggling with guilt and jealousy, to parents wrestling with responsibility, to grandparents suddenly changing their patterns with young ones, the disease hits hard across the entire family landscape. Events that once were simple—like going out to brunch or planning a family vacation—suddenly become a complicated task in diabetes management for the entire family. In each case, you need to consider each individual relationship to the child with the disease.

Sibling Matters

It's not easy having your sibling diagnosed with diabetes. First, your parents pretty much disappear into the hospital setting with your sibling. You wait that out and worry, thinking not only of your sibling's well-being but of your place in the family. When your brother or sister comes home, you expect it all to go back to normal. But suddenly, everything has changed. What's a kid to do? More to the point, what's a parent to do?

Attention Issues
Your child with diabetes will most likely be showered with flowers, gifts, cards, and sympathy. Everyone will reach out and let her know they care. This can be tough on a sibling. Even after a child comes home from

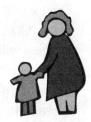

hospitalization, the gifts and attention can continue. While it's fine to let that happen, it is important to remind friends that your other children have been impacted by this disease as well.

You may want to give your other children a token of appreciation for the hardship they endured during diagnosis day. You'll also want to make sure, as time goes on, that your other children understand that diabetes does take up a lot of time and attention and that, in fact, the entire family is going to have to work toward a new normal.

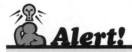

Alert!

At some point, you may need to ask friends to stop showering your child with diabetes with gifts. More than one parent has described this time as the "present-a-day program." You will have to move past overindulgence eventually, for everyone's sake.

That new normal may not be exactly what a sibling wants in life, and that needs to be discussed and understood early on. Sibling rivalry is natural in any family dynamic. In the case where a child gets added attention for any reason (and diabetes can be a big reason), parents need to point out to siblings that while added attention will go to the sibling with diabetes, it is the goal as a family not to take away attention from other siblings. A good first step toward helping a sibling understand that is acknowledging that so much attention is going to the other child. Talk about time and management issues right now ("We are still learning how to adjust insulin and may need to spend a lot of time on the phone with the doctors for a while"). Ensure that your other child will not be robbed of anything because of it. ("Of course I'll still be on the sidelines at all your tennis matches. Nothing will change that"). Point out to siblings that the simple things in life—youth sports, play dates, carpools—will not change for them; this realization will help them take a first step toward understanding where they fit into the picture.

Regression in Siblings

If you have a child who is younger than the child diagnosed with diabetes, don't be surprised to see a bit of regression. Diabetes is almost like a new baby coming into the house. It requires your attention, worry, and sleepless nights for a while. Children sense that and act out to try to grab your attention back. If you do see regression, take time to make sure you are truly giving your other child the same amount of attention you were before diabetes entered your life. It is easy for the parent or caregiver of the newly diagnosed to lose track of everything but managing the new disease. It's your responsibility not to lose track of your other children.

As time goes by, your other children are going to realize that, in fact, diabetes is not going away. While that's a big struggle for the child with diabetes to accept, it is also difficult for the siblings. It's a good idea for each parent to choose a "special event" each week with siblings: a long walk and an ice cream, or a movie date. Carve out a couple of hours each week to spend with them alone. Promise to do this and keep to it.

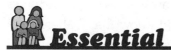

Essential

It's okay to celebrate milestones in your family's new life with diabetes. Some families even hold a "diagnosis day" party each year. Just remember to shower siblings with gifts and special attention on that day as well.

In the end, there is no avoiding giving your child with diabetes the lion's share of attention. But if you can back that up with a true effort to help siblings understand and still feel equally appreciated, you'll go a long way toward avoiding jealousy and anger issues.

Worries and Fears

Siblings harbor their share of worries and fears as well. Why did this happen? Will my sister die? Will it happen to me? More questions than parents can even imagine swirl through even the youngest (or most mature) minds. It is important to give each child a forum to air those fears and questions and to give them real answers.

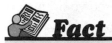 **Fact**

> Many siblings are fearful just from the name of the disease, thinking they hear DIE-abetes. Tell siblings right away that their brother is not going to die from diabetes and that you are learning to take good care of him.

Children will hear a lot of talk around their sibling's diagnosis and may be subject to such insensitive lines as "My great aunt lost her leg to diabetes," or, "Too bad, if he'd just kept away from sugar." Address these topics ahead of time. Let each child know that diabetes is a treatable disease and that the type her brother has is not the result of poor diet or bad life management. In simple terms, tell her that her brother's body stopped making insulin and you are learning how to help give it the insulin it needs. Give her response lines to store for such moments, such as "My brother has Type 1 and that is different," or "Diabetes is easier to treat today with the new tools."

What about the one question that comes most often and cuts to the heart of siblings: "Does it run in the family?" (See Chapter 1 for details on who gets diabetes and why.) It is crucial to tell your child from the start that while there are some rare cases where siblings also develop Type 1 diabetes, in almost all cases, they do not. Type 1 diabetes does not run in families; there is only about a 2 to 5 percent risk of carrying it over to a sibling. Your child needs to hear that from you (and it might be best to say there is a 95 percent chance they will *not* get the disease).

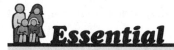 **Essential**

Show, don't just tell. Use diagrams and books, such as *Taking Diabetes to School* by Kim Gosselin (one of the best children's books describing diabetes on the market), to explain diabetes to your other children. Find pictures, posters, and other things to help siblings visualize and understand diabetes.

For families who want to know, there are studies that can detect whether siblings carry the antibodies for possible development of diabetes. The study, called TrialNet (*www.diabetestrialnet.org*), looks for three different antibodies in a child. Although it can tell you that a child may develop diabetes, it cannot tell you with all certainty that a child will or will not.

Siblings will also be afraid that your close tie to the child with diabetes means that you will love their brother or sister more. Promise them on a regular basis that you'll carve out time that is theirs and theirs alone.

Extended Family

At the start, grandparents, aunts, uncles, and other close relatives, for the most part, know just what to do: send gifts and warm thoughts. But once you get home and life begins again, oftentimes extended family members have a hard time figuring out what to do next. Many are afraid—of needles, of highs and lows, and of making some kind of mistake while the diagnosed child is in their care. This fear can cause some extended family members to back off.

The Need for Family Help

Ironically, there is no time in life a parent needs the support of their parents and relatives more. Asked what would make dealing with the diagnosis of their child easier from the start, many parents answer that having an extended family member totally on board would change their life for the better.

But it's hard. First of all, diabetes and kids is a complicated combination. Just look at all you had to learn in the hospital. How can an extended family member expect to catch on to all of that? The simple answer is that you must invite them to do so. While in your grief and worry, you may think family members are letting you down, in fact, they may think you don't believe that they are educated enough about diabetes to help. So as you learn, allow loved ones to learn as well.

 ## Essential

The Barton Center for Diabetes Education in North Oxford, Massachusetts, holds an annual Caretakers Weekend. Your child with diabetes attends with a grandparent or other caretaker, and the loved one comes back knowing how to care for her around the clock. For more information, visit ✍ ww.bartoncenter.org.

Some families who successfully integrate grandparents, aunts, and uncles into daily living with diabetes do it in the most obvious way: The relatives spend a lot of time just hanging around and watching. Ask your relative to come over each day for a week before breakfast, then before lunch, then at snack time, then at dinner, then at bedtime. By watching you develop your routine with your child, they'll develop into it as well.

Distance Matters

Of course, this is only possible if you live nearby. For relatives who live farther away, education can be more challenging. Such relatives should be encouraged to read up on Type 1 diabetes and children, and to visit Web sites for information, support, and feedback from others in their position. Encourage distant relatives to make a long-term visit to you (particularly grandparents). A solid week spent with you and your child will teach them much about life with diabetes.

Another good idea in this time of high-speed communication is to start a family diabetes blog. Your blog can talk about days in your child's life with diabetes, offering tips and useful information. As you develop the blog, you will also be creating a database of your own information. Relatives across the world can log on, learn, and feel as if they're helping you and caring for your child.

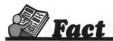 **Fact**

Caregivers who have the help and support of their parents report adapting to life with diabetes much quicker than others. Being able to trust someone else with your child is a giant step toward your new normal, and your parent is the perfect first person.

You may also want to suggest that your parents and relatives attend a support group meeting with you or, better yet, one of your endocrinology appointments. Don't overcrowd a room, but consider bringing one key support person each time for the first few times you attend such events.

When Relatives Don't Want to Help

What about the relative who just does not want to help out? It happens, and there can be many reasons. Many people are simply too afraid of diabetes to learn more about it. If some of these people happen to be your relatives, it can be hurtful. You, as a parent, may feel abandoned in your time of need.

The best thing to do is to address the family member in a non-confrontational way. Tell her that you've noticed she's backed away from spending time with your child. Assure her that you were afraid at first, too, but with education, she can go back to those sleepovers or play dates your child used to love so much. Offer to stay close by the first few times the relative attempts to care for your child.

If even this does not work, it's time to accept that you are not alone. More than a few parents say they have no help outside of their own home. Perhaps some good friend will jump on board and learn all about caring for your child so you can have some backup, some freedom, and, most of all, some compassionate support.

Spouses and Sharing the Disease

The diabetes diagnosis can be the ultimate bond and then, in time, the ultimate divider for parents. In the first days, parents share their grief, fears, and worries, leaning on each other to get themselves—and their child—through that difficult time. But it's easy for all that to fade and fade fast. Once home, one parent (often the mother) becomes the dominant care provider. It is all too easy, at that point, for the two parents to assume separate roles.

When Did I Become June Cleaver?

Mothers who had long considered themselves equals in every way to their spouses often find after diagnosis that they slip into more of a stereotypical parenting role, assuming most of the responsibilities while Dad takes on fewer hands-on duties. This happens in even the most balanced and close-knit families for one simple reason: Taking care of a child with diabetes can be nearly all-consuming. The parent who spends more time at home with the child (again, more times than not, the mother, but certainly there are fathers who do so as well) tends to climb the learning curve quicker, leaving the other parent in the dust.

In time, it just becomes easier to hand off diabetes duties to that dominant parent, and suddenly, the dominant parent feels truly alone in the battle. "All I need are pearls and an apron!" one mother, a part-time attorney, lamented at a support group nearly a year after her son was diagnosed. "How did I become June Cleaver?"

In most cases, the parents have passively allowed this to happen. It takes communication, understanding, and sometimes, giant steps backward to correct this situation.

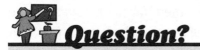

Question?

What if I just don't trust my spouse or partner?
If this is the case, for your child's sake, you need to ask your medical team to plan a training session for you and your spouse to bring you both to a level of agreement on shared care. This must be a team effort, and your child must see it as that.

Think of this new time in your relationship as crucial. In life, it is the challenges that make us stronger and bring us closer together— or tear us apart. While it may be hard for you to accept that your spouse forgets to wipe a finger with a swab before a finger stick or counts your child's carbs a little off, it is important for your child to feel safe (and loved) with both of you.

The Dominant Caregiver

It happens in almost every family. One parent, usually the one with the most flexible schedule, becomes the dominant parent in the diabetes care equation. As that parent grows stronger and more confident in her knowledge, the other parent tends to step back, allowing the spouse to take over. This is natural. First, who really wants the responsibility of caring for a child with diabetes 24/7? Almost anyone would admit that if they could avoid it, they would. Second, the breadth of knowledge necessary to care for a child with diabetes is almost endless. No parent just checking in part-time could possibly compete eye-to-eye with the fully educated parent.

Sharing the Disease

So what's a couple to do? It's clear that couples who, from the beginning, share in as much of the education as possible, fare better in this situation. If you can, make a commitment for both parents to attend every endocrine-type appointment for the first year of the child's diagnosis. Much of the learning goes on during that first year, so even if the second parent does not have as much hands-on experience, he or she will have been in on all the official medical discussions surrounding the child's care.

You'd be surprised how many couples don't follow that simple concept. With work demands, a limited number of sick days, and often a hearty drive to the pediatric endocrinologist, it's easy for full-time working parents to trade off on appointments, or for the parent who doesn't work or who works part-time to shoulder all the responsibility. This first, basic step will go a long way to keeping both parents on a somewhat level playing field.

The Passive Caregiver

The willingly passive parent has some kind of fear: of needles, of hurting her child, of accepting the reality of having a child with an incurable disease. Often, the passive parent is avoiding reality. While it's impossible for the dominant parent to push the reality on to the passive parent, it's a good idea to find a constructive way to bring her on board.

"If I were hit by a truck, what would happen?" More than a few dominant parents have lamented. The answer is simple and telling: The passive parent would learn to cope. The lesson here is that both parents need to come to a middle ground. The parent in charge all the time needs to know that she can count on her spouse when she needs a break. The passive parent needs to know that if he doesn't do everything exactly the same way the dominant parent does, he won't be lectured or criticized. Finding that balance, a place where both parents and their own diabetes care style can coexist in a non-confrontational and trusting way is a giant step toward helping your family live a healthy life with diabetes.

The Middle Ground

It's a good idea for parents who work long hours to try to find a way to have hands-on care. If you have weekends off, make Saturday and Sunday your diabetes care days. Take on all the responsibility those days. The spouse who usually has that care needs to let it go. Be available for discussion, but let your spouse live and learn the same way you are living and learning. It will only take a few weekends of constant care for Dad to begin seeking information about daily care topics. Getting that time off will free up Mom to think about other things, and possibly learn more about diabetes complications and research (or just get a pedicure).

In the end, the balanced family—with parents who share knowledge and understanding, who both can give great care to their child in a pinch; and with siblings who understand diabetes issues and still feel attended to—is the best environment for a child with diabetes.

What about Us?

The one thing that can get lost quickly in the shuffle of life with diabetes is any semblance of a romantic relationship. Quite like when a new baby comes home, the newly diagnosed child can not only take up a lot of your time and thoughts but also can make a couple feel incapable of leaving the house together. Some couples report waiting more than a year before having the nerve to go out on a date and leave their child with a sitter. Others never do.

 Essential

Do not make the assumption that all babysitting duties should go to an older sibling. Only opt for this if the older sibling is interested in taking on the duty. Some siblings feel bitter at being forced into this caretaking role and not being asked or appreciated.

Getting the guts to go out together as soon as possible will accomplish two important goals: reminding you that you are, indeed, a couple and proving to your child that life can and will go on as almost normal.

Many parents are not comfortable with the average thirteen-year-old girl around the corner for babysitting once diabetes enters their lives. If you do not have a family member willing to be trained in the basics, you need to figure out how to get a sitter you can trust.

In a perfect world, the teenager down the block was diagnosed five years earlier and you call on them (okay, in a perfect world, there is no diabetes, but we digress). Apart from this kind of luck, how does a parent find good babysitting care? Turn to your resources. First, try word of mouth. Have other parents in your town heard of older kids with diabetes you could call? Is there a commuter nursing student around who might need to make extra cash? Could your school nurse pass your name on to an older child with diabetes? You can also try to find a teen through your local diabetes support groups, or ask your local high school to allow you to post a want ad on the bulletin board.

Settle for Less than Perfect

But here's another thought: You don't need to have perfect, fully trained care. In this era of cell phones and instant access, parents should feel comfortable heading out for dinner or a movie for a few hours. Time your date to begin just after a shot (if your child is not on a pump) and then call to check in at blood check time. Or better yet, ask the sitter to send you the number on your handheld PDA. If it's within a decent range, order another glass of wine and relax. Getting out as a couple will remind you that you do have a life outside diabetes. No matter how hard it is the first time, dig deep and just do it. Your relationship, your family, and your child will thank you for it.

Divorced Parents and Diabetes Planning

As if it weren't hard enough to balance life with diabetes, divorce can double the challenges. Divorced parents, no matter how amicable or angry, will need to put aside their personal hurt and work as a team to make life work well for their child with diabetes as he travels between the two homes. And parents will be challenged: The trauma of the diagnosis can bring back hurt and anger from the past that just don't need to be revisited now.

Two Homes, One Plan

Hard as it may be, you will need to come up with a plan that works in harmony with both homes. First, every diabetes supply your child needs for any reason will need to be stored at each home. Talk to your medical team about making sure your prescriptions cover enough to keep stocked in two places. Toting it all back and forth is too much to expect, and things would be forgotten. You should set a planned date each month when the parent who is in charge of refills delivers supplies to the other. Don't waver from that date any more than you would from a child-support payment or a visitation drop-off or pickup.

As hard as it may be, parents will also need to attend all the medical appointments together. This can get a bit crowded. If there are stepparents involved, you'll need to talk to your medical team about making sure every parent can be a part of the ongoing medical education without overwhelming the room. You may need to appoint a parent to take notes and share with other stepparents, if the medical team asks that you limit the number of people who attend.

 Essential

The only absolute for divorced parents should be the "one logbook" rule. Parents should either share a logbook online or hand one back and forth for visitations. This way, everyone can see the entire picture of the child's week and all the child's information remains on the same page.

Parents should also be sure to share any pertinent information about the child's week when handing off for visitations (e.g., "Suzy had a minor stomach bug last night," or "Billy played four hours of lacrosse today").

Don't Be a Disney Dad or Mom

Even if you have long been the fun parent in the divorce situation, now is the time to understand that you simply cannot waver from the standard of care that your diabetes team has set up for your child. Come to an agreement as parents on what food and activity choices are acceptable. Don't let your child break rules that are set at one home. You should never hear, "At Mom's house I never have to wear my medic alert when I go out and play!" Do not ever question your ex's diabetes care choices to your child. Children have a way of finding things to use to manipulate situations. Even suggesting to your child that her diabetes care could be a weapon she could use against either of you is a dangerous precedent to set. Hard as it may be, wait until a private time, either on the phone, in person, or via e-mail, to discuss any concerns you may have with your ex.

Nobody's Perfect

At the same time, be reasonable in your expectations. No one is perfect. If your child comes home having missed a few blood checks or run a few highs, discuss the situation quietly and privately with your ex. And remember, you're not perfect either. If you begin to see patterns that concern you, and your ex does not respond in a cooperative way, discuss this with your child's social worker. Often, a third party can find a middle ground that can work for all of you.

What if your ex simply does not care well for your child? Then, you have a larger situation on your hands. In that case, it is most likely time for some professional intervention, such as a family counselor or your medical team. Remember, your child's future is more important than your personal needs.

When Diabetes Strikes More Than One Child

It's rare and the odds are low (again, about 5 percent), but it happens. When a second child (and in very rare cases, a third child) is diagnosed with diabetes, the family has to adapt all over again. While people seem to think that it is not as big of a deal as the first diagnosis, the second, in fact, can be even more devastating and take even more work to adapt.

Diagnosis Day

In most cases, a second child's diabetes is caught much sooner. Parents are all too familiar with the signs of high blood sugar (frequent urination, bedwetting, weight loss, excessive thirst) and also are extremely sensitive to watching for it in their children without diabetes. The good news is that many children don't go to the point of a medical crisis before diagnosis, since parents pick up on the signs and usually check the child's blood sugar early on.

When a second child is diagnosed, most parents call their primary care physician and ask to be referred directly to their endocrinology team. At this time, not all children need to be treated as inpatients, although some are.

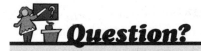 *Question?*

Would there be any benefit to having my second child treated as an inpatient?
Some parents find that, because of the shock of the moment, it's better to have a child stay at least twenty-four hours as an inpatient. This gives your medical team time to assess what the initial doses should be and give your child a chance to adapt. Other families prefer to do that from home.

Whether you choose for your child to be treated inpatient or out, you need to accept one fact quickly: Every diabetes case is different and every child reacts to insulin, food, and exercise in his own unique way.

Separating the Issues

Immediately, you need to set up a way to keep each child's diabetes in its own world. You may need different types of insulin, different supplies, and certainly a different logbook. By setting each up using color coding or in separate drawers or shelves, you won't mix them up (that often).

Remember, too, that this is your second sibling's own personal experience. Just because your first child diagnosed gave himself shots right off does not mean your second child will. Just because your second child wants to find a different endocrinologist doesn't mean your first has to as well. Each child needs, and requires, his own parameters for dealing with the disease.

Guilt and the First Child

It will be important to let your first diagnosed child know she had nothing to do with this second diagnosis happening. Some children can think it's their fault, that they are the ones who "brought diabetes into the house." Talk about these misconceptions; put them to rest once and for all.

The first child may also experience a tiny bit of jealousy. For years, the family-walk team shirts have been screened with her face; now she'll share that spot with her brother. For months, he's been the one who has been uniquely brave in the family; now he's got company. Be sure to remind your first diagnosed child of the fear he felt in those early days, and point out why you may need to give some extra help to your second child for a while. If you've had a special routine with the first child on appointment days (say, you always went to the appointment and then out for a one-on-one special lunch), find a way to keep that tradition without having to double your doctor visits.

CHAPTER 10

School Time

N ext to home, school is the place your child spends the most time and expects to feel most comfortable. School is the first big challenge to families adapting to life with diabetes. Parents want to create a situation where their child is safe, well cared for, understood, and most of all, treated like an equal. A good, seamless school plan is a must for childhood success living with diabetes.

The First Day Back

If your child is diagnosed during the school year, you (and your child) are not going to want to miss a beat. Sometimes, this will mean that a morning after returning home from an inpatient experience, you have to send your child off into the world without you. First days back to school can be worrisome for parents, for children, and for school officials. You and your child have not settled into your diabetes routine yet. You're barely getting a grasp of his first set of doses, and he may not have even experienced his first low yet. But back to school he must go, and your first step is first-day planning.

The First Visit to the School Nurse

The nurse is going to be your friend for life. At least that's your hope. So the first thing you need to do when sending a child back to school is to meet first with your child and the school nurse. Let the nurse know that today, you're just setting up day-to-day parameters, and

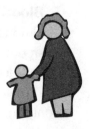

that a long-term plan will be worked out in the near future with your medical team's expertise, your expectations, and her assistance. For this first day, agree to times your child will check her blood sugar and how that will happen.

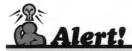

Alert!

No child of any age should ever head to the nurse's office to check on a low or high without someone accompanying him. Tell the nurse right away that your child must have a buddy with him for all nurse visits, so that your child is never walking alone to the nurse's office when high or low. You don't want your child to run into trouble along the way without someone to get help.

Bring with you vials of your child's insulin, syringes, a second meter to keep at school and test strips to go with it, a second ketone meter if you can get one (and ketone strips if you cannot), and depending on the size of your school, one or more glucagon kits to keep at school at all times. It's also a good idea to provide the nurse with a mini carbohydrate-counting directory. You can find one in the cookbook section of your local bookstore.

Ask the nurse to open the vials only when necessary, since they stay usable longer if they are unopened. You'll also want to provide the nurse and the classroom with their own supply of goodies to treat low blood sugar. Fill a plastic sealable container with individual bags of chips, crackers, and juice boxes, as well as a package of glucose tabs.

Blood Checks with the Nurse or in the Classroom

Although some students check their blood sugar levels in the classroom (more on that in the long-term plans section), most parents opt for their children to visit the nurse the first few days and even weeks. It's a good idea even if your child seems independent, if only to encourage a relationship between her and the nurse (something you'll cherish in time). These visits can also help the nurse get up-to-speed on diabetes and your child. The nurse will see what your child's plan and pattern is, how she deals with the new routine, and how she looks and feels during highs and lows. You're going to want this kind of relationship, even if your long-term plan is to have your child not visit the nurse as often.

Teacher in the Loop

What is the teacher's role during these first days? You'll need to sit down with him as well and go over a short-term plan for the first few days. The teacher will need to know that your child must be allowed to see the nurse, visit the restroom, or go for water at any time she requests. Point out to the teacher that you and your child are in a learning phase, and that the first weeks will be all about figuring things out. Ask the teacher to be part of the planning meeting you hold soon to develop a long-term diabetes plan for your child in school.

Some teachers will be fearful; others will be helpful. Encourage your teacher to share his honest concerns about your child and her diabetes. If you don't have good answers, promise to find them. A calm, involved teacher is best for your child.

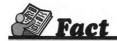 **Fact**

Most teachers will only have had past experiences with older relatives with Type 2 diabetes. Be sure, on the first day, to explain the vast difference between the two diseases, and remind the teacher that each child with diabetes is unique. This fact will help teachers not prejudge your child's care.

Your teacher will need to understand what times of day your child needs to eat and why. Some teachers will allow all students in their class to have an optional snack at the same time the child with diabetes has hers, often at 10 A.M. and 2 P.M. on the two-snack-a-day program. This solution helps the child feel "normal" and also reminds her to eat. If your child's teacher is willing to do this, suggest that class does not have to stop for this snack. Rather, students can be invited to eat a small snack as they continue their lessons.

How, When, and What to Tell Other Students

This is one of the biggest decisions you'll make in the first days. Most young children are happy to have you come in and help them tell their class what diabetes is and what it means, but older children can beg you to be secretive.

A simple rule is that the more people who know the better, and the earlier they know, the better it is for your child. This is true for a number of reasons. First, diabetes is a complicated and dangerous disease. The more people who know your child has diabetes and understands what that means, the safer your child is. Second, diabetes is nothing ever to be ashamed of or to hide from. While a child may claim he just wants privacy, allowing him to start out with a secret sends a dangerous subliminal message that there is some reason he should keep it to himself. Strongly encourage him to be as open about his diabetes from the start as possible.

Telling the News, Little-Kid Style

Smaller children are easy to work with on this. A good idea is to ask the teacher to let you and your child make a presentation that first day back. All the kids will know that your child was in the hospital and that something happened. By explaining what diabetes is and what it means for your child, the children will feel secure and will be able to help your child. Again, Kim Gosselin's book *Taking Diabetes to School* is magnificent in its simplicity and is the best way to get the message of diabetes across to teachers as well. Have your child read it to the class, and donate a few copies to stay in the classroom.

Allow the students to have a question-and-answer period after your presentation. You might be surprised at some of the questions that arise, and by addressing them, you can put a lot of misconceptions and questions to rest. Expect to hear "Can I catch it?" and "My grandpa had it." Respond in simple terms and on their level. There's no need for medical jargon here, obviously.

Telling the News, Older-Kid Style

With tweens (ages nine through twelve) and teens, it becomes more difficult to let the world know. Even for older kids, there have to be some minimum requirements. To start, every teacher the child deals with must be notified that your child now has diabetes. This is usually best done in a meeting (particularly in middle school) where teachers can ask questions and voice concerns.

Your child might not like this, but it's best for her that everyone knows what is going on. From there, it is up to your child how much she wants to share with other students. Some children this age feel comfortable presenting their disease and its details as an essay in English class or as a science fair project. Others would rather not discuss it in public. Talk to your child and with your medical team to develop a reasonable compromise.

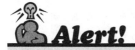

Alert!

Make sure your school places a small reminder card about your child's diabetes on every teacher plan book. That way, all substitute teachers will know about your child's medical situation and not be taken by surprise. Nor will your child have to explain.

In the end, the more open your child is willing to be in school about his diabetes, the better the situation is for everyone. In time, he should find that being open and honest about his diabetes will make for less talk, fewer whispers, and fewer questions in the future. Eventually, it will just become part of the school landscape and something everyone around him quietly knows.

Making the School Nurse Your Partner

In the first months and even for a long time after that, you can expect to speak to the school nurse on a regular basis. It is important, from the start, to develop a cooperative relationship, one in which your nurse lends expertise and support but understands that you and your medical team are in charge.

Your school nurse may or may not have had experience with other children with diabetes, and this experience may or may not be a good thing for you. While it's always good to have had another family blaze a trail for you, it is important for the school nurse to understand that your child's situation is unique. Encourage your school nurse to share with you any ideas or suggestions she's seen work, but remind her that your child needs to be cared for and treated in the way you and your medical team deem best, not in the way she may assume works because of her experience.

 Essential

Laws prohibit nurses from sharing medical information about other students, but they do not prohibit you from asking your school nurse to pass your phone number on to other parents. Use your nurse as a resource.

Once you and your child have settled in and survived the first days, you and your nurse will want to begin long-term plans for making your child feel comfortable and keeping her safe in school. Again, although you are leading, it is important that your nurse feel like a partner in the planning. By including him in discussions and ideas, and explaining with medical backup why you might ask that your child be treated differently from another child with diabetes, you'll have a better chance of keeping his respect and partnership.

One of the biggest decisions is training someone else to administer glucagon. In almost every case, schools prefer that only the nurse is trained. On a larger campus, however, you may want to try to convince the nurse to have a second person on the opposite side of the school trained as well. Ideally, this could be a vice principal or a guidance counselor. This issue should be part of the discussion when you work on your long-term plan.

Flow of Information

You and your nurse will want to figure out a way to share information on your child's diabetes without crossing any lines. Some parents are hesitant to share entire logbooks with nurses; they want to keep their home life and the totality of the disease private. Others don't mind sharing at all. It's your call. For the most part, nurses need to know how your child is doing during the school day and any information that pertains to that day (such as a low overnight, or a high early that morning). You and your nurse should come up with a way to share that information without having to spend all your time on the phone.

Some parents choose to send notes; others call the nurse on unusual mornings to discuss the upcoming day. Most parents opt to let the school nurse keep her own logbook and send their child home with numbers to record in the home logbook.

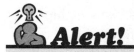

Alert!

E-mail is a great way to keep everyone in the loop. With more schools now online, nurses, teachers, and even students can now simply e-mail a blood sugar reading and send a copy of it to everyone involved. This makes the information accessible at all times.

Is there any information you don't have to provide to your nurse? Absolutely. Knowing overall readings, particularly for a younger child, can help a nurse; however, what is going on and possibly coming in the disease is your business. Should you allow a nurse to talk directly to the medical team? Most parents advise against it. Any situation that requires talking to the team should require talking to a parent as well. In this age of cell phones and wireless communication, seldom is there a time that a parent or guardian cannot be reached first.

504s and Other Long-Term Plans

Once you've settled in and bonded with the school nurse, it's time to think long term. You'll want to find a way not only for your child to settle in, but for you and your child (and your school) to be on the same page and not have to worry constantly about what comes next.

The 504

Your child will need a written set of rules and plans for his school day, usually in the form of a 504 plan. A 504 plan, named for the section it falls under in the Education Rehabilitation Act of 1974, is a plan for students who have special medical or educational needs in the school environment. Your child's diabetes means that, under federal law, you can set up certain things for her to ensure her safety and equal education each school day.

What do parents like to include in 504s? Obviously, you will include the basics. First, your child can take as many bathroom or water breaks, or visit the nurse as needed each day. Also, she can carry and eat snacks at any time. Many parents push for, and get, more. Some ask that a child be allowed to carry a meter in school and to check wherever he'd like.

Additions to the 504

The 504 plan can allow a child more absences than schools normally allow; it can also include how long a child has to make up work and provide for tutoring if a child misses many days. Aggressive plans can call for anything from carrying a cell phone in school (to call parents with blood sugar readings), to holding off on testing if blood sugar readings taken just prior to the exam are too low or too high, and, in one case, to providing a full-time aide trained in insulin-pump management to be placed in the classroom with a young child.

Set up your 504 meeting for a time that works for you, the teachers, the nurse, the principal, and the school psychologist. If possible, ask one of your medical team to draft a letter explaining your expectations and goals. When discussing your requests, always point out that you are asking the advice of your child's "medical team." In most cases, schools want to help a child come up with a plan that will mean academic success and social happiness.

Other Plans

What about testing, beyond what's laid out in the 504? It's a good idea to have a frank discussion with your child's teachers about low and high blood sugars and how they can impair cognitive reasoning. Most teachers have no idea that children with diabetes often experience huge blood sugar swings. Explain that this, sadly, is not out of the norm for a child with diabetes. Download some facts on lows, highs, and testing and share them with the teacher. In most cases, teachers truly care and will take that into account if an unusual low grade pops up in a student's portfolio. Some teachers even take the time to call a parent if a good student struggles on a test to make sure it was not a low or high blood sugar day. Sharing such concepts and making plans can only help your child.

What you don't need to worry about, for the most part, is that your child will use lows and highs as an excuse. Most children with diabetes do not want to consider themselves hampered by the disease. Most will never use it as an excuse. Let your teachers know that if your child says he's struggling with a blood sugar, he most likely is.

When Your School Doesn't Have a Nurse

Hard as it is to believe, some schools, even public schools, do not have a school nurse. Most parents or caregivers are frozen with fear at the idea of sending a child with diabetes to school without a nurse, but it can be done in a way that makes families feel safe.

Finding a Solution

If you are in this situation, you'll need to sit down with your school principal and possibly the district director of student services to talk about why a nurse is needed, and what you and the school will do to make your child safe without one. Some parents have moved their children to other schools that have nurses, but most parents don't want to disrupt their children's lives any more than they already have been.

If there is no school nurse, another adult in the school, usually a willing teacher or administrator, needs to learn all about your child's diabetes and be there as her support person during the school day.

Some schools scoff at this idea because of liability issues. Try to find other parents of children with diabetes who have made the situation work in their no-nurse school, and share their experience. Hope that your school staff will buy in. If they don't, you may need to consider asking them to allow your child to carry a cell phone and setting up set times during the school day when you or your spouse or another adult familiar with your child's care checks in with her.

Supply Management with No Nurse

Not having a nurse will mean you'll have to be even more careful to make sure your child's school supplies remain well stocked. Without a nurse to remind you, you can easily run out of snacks or insulin or lancets at school. Make a monthly visit to the school to check on your child's supplies, so he never falls short on something he needs. That's the funny thing about diabetes supplies: You never seem to need them until you don't have them within reach.

You'll also want to discuss with your school where your child's supplies will be kept. With no nurse's office, you'll need a cool and secure place to store them. If the school cannot provide this, you may need to consider a small fridge as a donation, just to keep your child's supplies correctly stored.

The Rest of the Team

You'll need everyone who oversees your child in school—from lunchroom aides to recess attendants to coaches to bus drivers—to understand your child's diabetes and be willing to watch out for her. Educating these supervisors from the start and giving them specific roles will only help and protect your child.

Bus Drivers

Particularly if your child has a long bus ride, your bus driver will need to be told exactly what it means to have Type 1 diabetes, what the signs of a low are, and what should be done with a low. While you should always make sure your child carries fast-acting glucose on the bus and at the bus stop, you may want to slip a tube of glucose tabs into the bus driver's glove compartment. Remind your child, and the driver, that they are there in case of an emergency. Encourage the bus driver to look closely at your child when she gets on the bus each day: Bus stop frolicking can cause lows, and the end of the day is a ripe time for lows as well.

Also remind the driver that while he may have a strict rule about eating on the bus, it may be necessary for your child to eat from time to time. Explain that eating is not a treat, but a treatment for your child. Show him your child's meter and tell him your child may check on the bus if she feels low and not to worry (your child will not remove the lancet on the bus; she will take it home in the lancing device).

Recess and Lunchtime Aides

This group may be overlooked by parents, and they can actually be quite helpful. Recess and lunch aides are adept at keeping a keen eye on a large group of children. Understanding your child's needs will help them keep her safe.

First, ask one lunch aide and one recess aide for each day to have the duty of always having glucose tablets in their possession. Tell your child who they are and that they'll always have glucose available for her. Remind recess aides that kids should never walk alone to the nurse to be treated for a high or low. They should send a buddy every time. The main duty of lunch aides should be to ensure your child eats what she needs to, and if she is on a pump, to ensure that she does the lunch bolus she is supposed to. This is a fine line since kids with diabetes, for the most part, hate being nagged. But let's say your child sees the nurse for a shot and is expecting to eat a sandwich, then decides not to. If an aide sees that the child did not eat, she can let the nurse know.

 Essential

> Basic brochures on how to understand highs, lows, and other diabetes basics in school are available through the Juvenile Diabetes Research Foundation at *www.jdrf.org*, or by calling 1-800-JDF-CURE. These brochures are a great, simple resource to help part-time staff build their knowledge.

By letting these school employees know how they can help, you can ensure that your child will be surrounded by support. By asking them to be sure to watch passively, you'll ensure that it's not an overbearing situation for your child. As children get older, they'll need this kind of support less and less. But throughout school, it's a good idea to let these folks know your child has diabetes. You don't ever want someone confused over what might be an emergency situation.

When a School Won't Cooperate

It happens. For whatever reason, there are schools and teachers and nurses and coaches who do not cooperate with the standard of care that the medical team and family have developed. Some base their policies on old information instead of on new technologies and treatments. Others believe that it is not in their contracts to provide the extra attention and care a child with diabetes can use during the school day.

Enlisting Help

If you do find yourself in that situation, you'll need to get help fast. Your first option is to find another family with a child with diabetes who has had a good experience. Often, one school in a district may be handling things well when another is not. Set up a meeting between principals and nurses of both schools and go over your requests. Sometimes, all it takes is another school's success to help a school come on board.

If that is not available or does not work, ask your medical team if they have anyone they can refer. An advocate is someone who understands the needs of a child with diabetes and is seen by the school as a true expert. While parents realize that they are experts as well, sometimes schools think that parents are being overprotective or are overreacting to situations with their children. An outside expert can go a long way toward providing help in that situation.

Enable Your School to Break New Ground

Diabetes care has changed so drastically in the past few years, and more changes are coming. Just a decade ago, most children were on two shots a day and were forced to eat only at set times and not at any other time. Before that time, children were on one shot a day, and it was thought that little could be done about fluctuating blood sugars. Because of this, ironically, it was easier to care for a child in school.

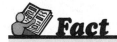 **Fact**

Younger kids in school on pumps are largely a product of the twenty-first century. Your child may, in fact, end up being the first child your school has ever had on an insulin pump. This first can be a good thing: You'll be the one setting the rules and making the procedures.

With the long-term advantages of tight control, better fast-acting insulin, and insulin pumps, there comes a bigger challenge in school.

Kids who run tight blood sugars are more apt to go low; kids who are on pumps can go high and spill ketones quicker. But in the school setting, it's a plus, because kids on tighter control feel better and do better in school.

Explain this to the staff at your school; show them studies. See if you can get them to embrace the idea of making your child's school experience with diabetes the most healthful and positive of this new era. Getting school staff to feel as though they're helping you be on the cutting edge of a better educational and social experience can go a long way. Win them over to your team. In the end, your child and the school will win.

CHAPTER 11

Playtime

P laytime is supposed to be carefree. Your smaller child heads out in the yard to frolic on the swings or sled down the back- yard hill. Your bigger kid wants to ride bikes around your quiet block. Your teen wants to hang at the beach or the mall. Playtime is supposed to be simply about fun, but for the parent of a child with diabetes, it is yet another moment of panic and concern. But with smart thinking, playtime can be fun again.

Around the Block Can Feel Like Around the World

With diabetes, the places you always felt were safe for your child sud- denly appear filled with new obstacles. Arranging playtime can be challenging, but with good planning, a well-thought-out approach, and notes to remind you how and when, you can once again send your child out to play safely, happily, and even if somewhat tethered to you, feeling almost free again.

Check Constantly (At First)

For the first few outings, you're going to need to be in information-gathering mode. Warn your child ahead of time. Let her know that the first few times she does any activity, as benign as it may seem, you're going to be a bit careful. Tell her you'll be checking her before she heads out and right when she comes in at the very least.

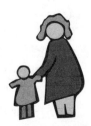

You may, if she is heading out for an extended period, need her to check her levels midway through the activity and give you a call, or if she is younger, she may need to meet you at some point and you'll check together. Let her know that this will not be forever. Eventually, you and your child will come to know, almost instinctively, how different activities affect her and what you need to do before and after them.

 Essential

Keep an activity logbook for the first year or so. Any time your child tries something new since his diagnosis, track his blood sugars, carbs consumed, time spent, and any reactions. You can refer back to your log for the second time, and in time, it will all just be backup material.

At the start, your child may balk at what she sees as an intrusion on her free time, so be sure to drive home the fact that, with information and in time, you'll be able to set her relatively free again. If she can see an end (of sorts) in sight, she may be more willing to react positively.

You may even want to go out of your way to have your child do some of his playtime activities a few times in the early months. The more you can get under your belt with a real-time understanding of what to expect blood sugars to do, the sooner you can give him a little bit more freedom. This activity might set your child free mentally too. Once diagnosed, some children can think that diabetes is going to limit them in activities and in life. Arranging an impromptu ski day (so you can see how that sport affects your child) can lead him to say, "Hey, I can still do everything I want."

Carry-alongs

It would be nice to be able to tell your child that she will never have to bring anything along with her as she plays, but the plain truth is she will need to. A general rule is the farther away she'll be playing, the more she'll need to bring.

Kids playing in your yard don't need to carry anything. You are there for them (or another caring adult is) if they need anything. But once they roam beyond that point, they need to pack backup supplies and carbs. It's not easy to carry a juice box, so glucose tabs or sweet candy like Skittles are best. This is a non-negotiable requirement for kids with diabetes who are out playing. Let your child know that if he is more than a few houses away from home and feels low, he should eat the carbs and should head home for a quick check. If he is wrong, it is better for him, in this case, to err on the side of caution.

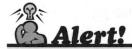

Alert!

Don't assume a snack or higher blood sugar just before heading out means your child does not need to be prepared. Lows are the result of how far and how quickly she drops, not necessarily to where she drops. In other words, a child who is 200 could feel low at 99.

It's a good idea to encourage your child to carry a meter if she is heading farther away than a few homes as well. This can seem inconvenient, but a child who is encouraged to stop and check when she is not feeling right is a child you'll be able to trust in the future. Find a way for her to carry her supplies easily. Some meters and lancet devices fit right into the zip pocket of a jacket (but be sure the pocket zips; more than a few meters have fallen out of the open pockets of playful children). Other devices fit into small backpacks if your child does not mind carrying one. If your older kid is heading farther away, this is non-negotiable. He simply must carry the tools he needs with him, and you cannot allow him to head far from home without a meter, strips, glucose, and a site change in case of emergency if he is on a pump. Expect a battle if your child is a teenager. Teens hate to be encumbered, but don't back down. The one time she needs it and doesn't have it, you'll regret it, and so will she.

Cell phones are the equivalent of the Apollo moon landing for playtime and kids with diabetes. A decade ago, some parents were astute enough to buy walkie-talkies for neighborhood play, but they had little way to keep track of kids who meandered farther. As much as you may not like the idea of giving a younger child a cell phone, you won't regret it. Insist that your child keep her cell phone on at all times while out playing. Promise that as time goes on you'll try *not* to check on her too often.

For younger kids, new cell phones that only allow them to call a few numbers are available. You may want to consider one for your own peace of mind.

What about medical alert jewelry? Little children, particularly girls, don't mind them at all, but older kids and boys can balk at them. Have your medical team back you up on this: When your child is away from you, wearing a medical alert piece is not negotiable.

Adjusting for Outside Days

Warm or cold, winter or summer, outside days are a whole different metabolic experience for kids with diabetes. The bad news is there is no set way of reacting to weather for all kids with diabetes. Some find cold makes them go low; others find blood sugars soar in the frigid air. Some children (many, really) find that heat and humidity seem to mean less and less insulin is needed; a rare few climb high on sticky days. Your challenge is to find out what different weather (and different levels of activity) means to your child. Again, it comes down to gathering data (blood checks), looking for patterns, and figuring out what happens to your child in these situations.

If It's Cold Outside

Winter, particularly frigid winters, can mean big changes for your child and his diabetes. First, there's the inactivity for much of the day. Cold, cold days can mean hours playing video games, reading, or watching television. If your child is relatively active, such a drastic change may cause some higher blood sugars. What's the right reaction?

Simple: Watch carefully for trends. One day of inactivity, if the weather looks better, should not mean a change in an insulin dose or basal rate. Look at it this way: If you change your child's basals or long-acting insulin doses based on one day's information, you'll be changing them every day, a near impossible situation. Rather, on such a quiet day, check a bit more often, and expect to do one or two correction shots or boluses. Remember, as long as you check, you can correct.

Then there is the cold active day. Most parents or caregivers will tell you: There's something about sledding that just drags that blood sugar down. Whether it's the trudging up and down the hill, the surge of endorphins while flying downhill, the cold air, or the drastic change from sitting inside, most parents find that sledding means an extra snack or two.

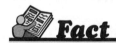 **Fact**

Meters don't always behave in the cold. Read your meter manual for details on what temperature it works best in. If your child is going to be outside for an extended time, make sure you take precautions to keep that meter warm enough to work correctly.

Your best bet on the first day out is to err on the side of caution. If your child's blood sugars are toward the low side of normal, you may want him to eat a small snack. If, in an hour or so, sledding does drop his blood sugar, he'll be thrilled to take a hot chocolate break without a shot or bolus. In time, the hot chocolate/snack break could become a happy part of your child's winter outdoor play expectations, and you can rest easy with the special snack, knowing the energy burned out in the cold makes it a necessary event. If your child is pumping, read your manual for details on what temperatures are of concern. Then purchase some kind of neoprene fanny pack–type device (available on pump accessory sites) for your child to put his pump into, and then have him place it under at least one layer of clothing. It will stay warm, toasty, and fully functional there, and not get in the way of winter fun.

If It's Hot Outside

And then there is the sweltering heat of summer (or for those who live in the South, most of the year). Families in more seasonal climates find that the change in insulin need from cold to warm can be almost shocking. Perhaps it is the extra activity that keeps children outside more, the longer days that mean they are more active or the effect of heat on the body, or a combination, but summer weather usually means cutbacks in insulin needs.

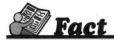 **Fact**

Insulin does not stand up well to heat. If you are carrying it with you, you must store it in a small cooler or cold space. Check out diabetes supply sites for small insulin coolers for such days.

Your first summer, it's a good idea to be on your toes. Talk to your medical team and see if they want to cut back on a dose or basal rate right from the get-go or if they'd rather wait and see how your child does.

If they choose the latter course, hot weather is a time to make doubly sure you are up to speed on blood sugar readings and have fast-acting snacks within reach. If your child is small, the first days of summer, with you hanging on and watching her every move, won't be a big deal. Just bring a logbook, take extra blood sugar readings, and track how things go. Have this information gathered after a couple of days of summer and call your medical team to discuss any summer dose/basal changes. If your child is older, hanging around with her and gathering information all day might be a problem. Explain that you want her to be able to live her usual summer life with all this new responsibility, but you need to help her figure out how. Remind your child that, like any other responsibility she has in life, readings must be adhered to in order to keep freedom.

Youth Sports and Diabetes

Youth sports are as ubiquitous to childhood today as Hula-Hoops were when today's parents were kids. It's hard to find a child who isn't involved in youth soccer, T-ball, Little League, gymnastics, or any other sport. Most children have a sport for every season, most social situations are centered around these activities. While managing your child in sports situations will take some time, you'll want to make it happen for them as soon as possible.

Coach on Board

Although by now you feel as if you've met with everyone on the planet, it is not the time to keep quiet when it comes to youth sports. It is your responsibility to tell your child's coach about her diabetes and to help him understand it. With the parents of your child's friends, you want to make sure the environment is safe for your child. With sports, your goal is simple: Help the coach understand that your child can be treated in the same way as any other player.

In the past, people thought that diabetes spelled the end of an athlete's competitive life. When Olympic champion (and fastest swimmer in the world) Gary Hall was diagnosed with Type 1 diabetes, his doctors and his coaches assumed he'd never compete again. Hall had the wherewithal to go out and find a new doctor, who helped him teach his coaches that diabetes does not mean the end of competition and sports. You may need to do the same thing with your child's coach.

After you sign your child up for the team and you're feeling a bit ill because you had to check yes under medical issues, call the league immediately and ask to set up a preseason meeting with the coach. This meeting should go over what it means for your child—on the field and the bench—to compete with diabetes. You'll want to put the coach at ease. Explain that you will monitor your child's blood sugar before (and sometimes during) games. Let her know that your child may need to eat on the sidelines and definitely needs to stay hydrated. Most of all, ask the coach to treat your child just as she would any other child on the team. Diabetes is not an indicator of athletic ability.

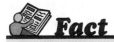 **Fact**

Go to ✏ *www.jdrf.org* and search for "athletes with diabetes." You'll find photos, bios, and tips from some famous jocks. Your child will be able to see that having diabetes does not mean that he or she can't excel in sports and fitness.

Game Day

It would be nice to know exactly how it is going to go every time your child competes, but part of the excitement of sports is the unknown. This means that your game plan will have to be flexible.

Obviously, you are going to check blood sugars before any competition begins, but what are you looking for? A good rule is to expect your child to go into the game a bit above what you consider normal range. If your daily goal is not to go over 150, starting a game at 200 is fine. If your child's lower range is not to be below 80, and he is, say, 90 at game start, it's a good idea to give him some carbs to boost him up a bit.

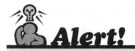

Alert!

A red flag for absolutely not playing in a game or match is the presence of ketones. When ketones are in the bloodstream—no matter what her blood sugar level is—exercise can definitely make it worse. This is one time you must say no, unequivocally, to your child's participation.

As for planning for actual playing time, don't. Too many parents have bulked their kids up on carbs only to see them sit on the bench or pumped in extra insulin only to see them play for the entire game. Be fluid. That's sports.

Safe Playgroups and Play Dates

What child doesn't like to play at a friend's house? His toys always seem more interesting, his mom serves different snacks, and your child feels as if he's on some kind of big-kid adventure. After diagnosis, parents struggle with the concept of playgroups and play dates, and many opt, at the start, simply to have them all at their home or insist on hanging around at them when they are elsewhere. The first option is not a good long-term one. Even the smallest child needs to know that she can be safe outside her own home, and needs to explore social situations outside her usual parameters. The second option, particularly with tiny tots with diabetes, is not outrageous. But in time, every parent should work toward finding a way to let his child visit and play with friends all by himself.

Playgroups

If your smaller child was in a playgroup before diagnosis, keep that as part of her life right from the time you come home. Most likely, you've bonded with the parents or caregivers in this group, so they may be a great first chance for you to educate others on diabetes and what it means for your child. The first few times your child attends, even if it is a drop-off group, ask to stay behind and show the host parent exactly what you do to care for your child during that time. Encourage her to learn how to do a blood check on your child; show her exactly what is used to treat a low and discuss good snack choices.

Then consider asking everyone to your house for a special play-group day. While the children play, do a mini-diabetes 101 program for the parents. Outline what it is and what it means to your child's day. Speak in positive terms: Help the parents feel comfortable with your child in their home. In most cases, other parents want to help you and your child live a normal life.

Play Dates

The phone rings, and it's the mother of the little boy your son recently met on the playground. They seemed nice and your children really hit it off. They want your son to come over and play (and ask if you can drop him off). While the natural instinct of the protective diabetes mom is to say no, you need to work toward a way you can just say yes.

On the phone, ask the mother if she knows your child has Type 1 diabetes. Explain that, when you arrive, you will need about ten minutes just to go over a few things, such as what your child needs to eat while there and at what time. Try to pick a time that works around shots or even blood checks, and take it from there.

When you arrive, have your child's snack schedule written down, and at least the first time, bring along a snack for your child and one for the host child. Tell the parent in no uncertain terms that your son must eat that snack at the specified time.

Just Say No

What if you just don't get a good feeling about a parent? If your instinct says no, you need to act the same way you would in any other potentially dangerous situation with your child. Offer for the other child to play at your house, but tell the other parent you just cannot send them over there. Like a house with unlocked guns or a parent who does not watch small children carefully, safety must come first.

Birthday Parties

Not long ago, parents had to scrape frosting off cupcakes and carefully weigh pieces of cake, but today, with the advent of short-acting insulin, birthdays can be much more carefree for kids, even if it does mean (as always) more work for the parents.

Treat Central

Birthdays seem to be all about the treats, from pizza to ice-cream sundaes to that always heralded cake. The best way to deal with this with your child is to plan ahead. Call the parent planning the party and discuss what he is planning on serving. Take notes, then crack open your carb list book, look up each item, and make a list to bring with you.

Some parents choose to give their child a bolus or shot and let them graze throughout the party, checking them when it ends to make any corrections that might be needed. Others like to keep track as the child eats ("Suzy? Is that your eighth chip or your ninth?"). A good solution is often somewhere in the middle. If the party is going to be a lavish buffet of foods you know your child cannot resist, do a half bolus to start things out and add another bolus or shot later on in the event. That way, if your child opts not to eat as much, you won't be in the tough spot of force-feeding them to match the insulin on board.

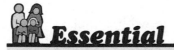 **Essential**

For any party your child is a guest at, offer to bring along Jell-O Jigglers. They're sugar free, brightly colored, and yummy. Most kids will go for them first, and they require no thought at all. You'll find the recipe on the side of the box of Jell-O.

When it comes to the cake, you'll want your child to eat just as any child would: not too big a piece, but not a tiny piece either. Don't be surprised if your child doesn't finish it. Often the games and fun distract the child from the very thing you stressed about the most. Do not scrape off the frosting or deny your child the cake. He needs to be treated like other kids, and you can always give more insulin if he really enjoys the cake.

Loot Bags: The Gift That Keeps on Giving

What party doesn't end with a loot bag nowadays? Most have some great prizes; almost all are crammed full of candy. Here is a place you can allow your child to be "different." Ask the host parent, in advance, not to give your child a loot bag full of candy. Sure, your child can eat candy, but stickers or pencils or the like are just as fun and less intrusive. Sometimes, the host parent will take a cue and give nonfood loot bags to everyone. Cross your fingers and hope that you're dealing with one of them.

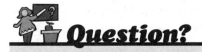 *Question?*

Should I ask the host to give my child sugar-free candy?
No. Remember that sugar-free candy has carbohydrates in it, too, and also requires carb counting and added insulin. Be sure to tell your host so they don't go to the trouble of purchasing special candy.

If you do find your child comes home with a sack of candy, suggest you keep it in the fridge, and remind your child that he needs to let you know when he is eating a piece. Consult your carb-counting book for counts on all candy; even little pieces have some carbs. You can also keep that candy in your low treatment supply, and offer your child something other than a glucose tab from time to time.

When You Are the Host

Talk to your child about her birthday party. Does she want to do it the way she did it before diabetes? If yes, plan it out. Figure out the amount of carbohydrates in a piece of cake, and cut every child's piece to that size. Then you'll know your child's carb count without even a thought. Give out a food-free loot bag and watch: Everyone will love it (even parents of kids without diabetes hate taking all those sweets home).

The Beach, the Mountains, and the Wilderness

If you love adventure and the outdoors, diabetes doesn't need to slow you or your child down. With good planning and the right tools, a day at the beach can be just that, and a trip to the mountains can still be a peak experience.

The Beach and the Water

It is tough enough getting sand in your flip-flops, so how do you manage diabetes in a beach setting? It's not easy, but it can be done. For boys and girls, the issue of how to carry along a meter and backup snacks is always difficult. No kid today wants to lug a pack around all the time, but he does need to have his items handy.

When your child heads to the beach, suggest that she and her friends set up a central spot for the day. They can spread their towels out, set down their other stuff, and your child can put down her supplies. Boys can tuck meters and insulin into the huge pockets of the shorts they wear over their bathing suits. Remind them that direct sunlight and heat can hurt their meter and damage the insulin, so they need to wrap their shorts in a large towel and store it somewhat in the shade. Girls may be willing to carry a cute beach bag–type purse, but again, it will need to be protected from the sun.

In a best-case scenario, your child is willing to carry a cooler to the beach and leave it with her towels. You can make this more palatable. Consider packing a cooler for *all* their friends. Fill it with flavored waters, fruits, and other fun beach snacks. When your child grimaces at having to bring the cooler, her friends will beg for it, making it okay and totally cool to bring it along.

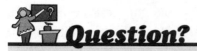

Question?

Can a beach day be a day off from diabetes?
Not completely, but in time, you can hedge. While there is never a time your child can just forget about his diabetes, he can, in good times, not check it for four to five hours. Only allow this once in a while though.

Pump It Up, Beach Style

What about wearing a pump on the beach? Most pumps are waterproof or at least water resistant now, so getting them wet is not an issue. But getting sand in the site and leaving them sitting on a towel can be problems.

Girls can be particularly picky about pumps with their teeny-tiny bathing suits, but the fact is, while they are at the beach (other than when swimming) they need to keep it on to make the day work well. Most girls choose a site on their hip or side of their leg for a beach day, and then they can tuck the pump into the side of their suit bottom without tubing flowing all over their bodies. Another good spot to tuck a pump is in the center of the back strap of the bikini top. Girls find that location works well with a belly site.

Little girls can follow that same plan, or parents can purchase waterproof neoprene cases that they can wear to hold their pumps. For boys, it's a bit simpler. Pumps can be clipped on the waistline of their bathing suit, or even in the pocket of suits that have them.

To Disconnect or Not?

When it comes to jumping in the water, most kids choose to disconnect. It's not that the pump might be in danger; it's more a question of comfort. While playing and splashing in the water, most children, particularly older children, would rather feel unencumbered. If you are not with them, you need to set strict rules about how the pump is stored while they are in the water.

First, purchase some high-quality zippered bags that you know will seal, and send them along with your child in the cooler. When your child is going to hit the waves, they should disconnect, store the pump in the bag, and place the bag in a secure, cool place.

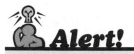

Alert!

Never leave a pump just sitting out in clear view. This is more than about keeping it cool. Pumps, which can be confused for iPods or pagers or video games, have been stolen—and as most families find out, insurance usually does not cover a new one.

If your child is in the water for a long period or wants to be disconnected, set some ground rules. A pump does not need to be on all day. Some children who are on swim teams stay disconnected for hours and hours. The key is you need to check more often. As long as your child checks her blood sugar every couple of hours, she can click the pump on and quickly administer any bolus that might be needed at that time, and she should maintain reasonable numbers all day.

On the Mountains

Skiing, snowboarding, and winter hiking affect different children in different ways. One girl, a beginner skier, reported her blood sugars soaring every time she hit the slopes. Her parents wrote it off to stress and learned to up her basals every ski day. Another girl, a lifelong skier diagnosed when she was a good five years into the sport, found she needed much less insulin on ski days and was able to take snack breaks without bolusing each ski day. It's all as unique as the pattern of each snowflake. Your job is to learn what your child's pattern is and make it work.

It's a good idea to spend the first day out with your child. Take your time and check a lot. Watch what the day does to your child. With that background, you can dive into your winter season with confidence.

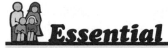

Essential

You'll want to stock your child's pockets with easy-to-eat snacks in case of chairlift or mountaintop lows. Try granola bars, which tend to not freeze, and easy-to-use glucose tabs.

While cell phones are your saviors everywhere else, reception can be spotty in the mountains. Good two-way phones are cheap now, and some resorts even rent them out of their ski rental shop. This precaution will give you, and your child, a sense of security, even if you barely use the phone.

The Wilderness

Camping and hiking don't have to end. You just have to be prepared. When heading out into the wilderness, pack two more of every diabetes supply item than you need. Backup meters are a must, as are multiple bottles of insulin (you never know when you might drop one). If your child is pumping and you will be far from civilization, call your pump company. Often, for special trips, pump companies offer loaners for you to carry in case a pump malfunctions.

You'll also want to pack plenty of carbs. Fish from a stream is lovely, but your child needs carbs to match her insulin each day. Granola bars and other energy bars are a great choice.

Making the effort to make these playtimes happen will send your child—and the world—a powerful message: Kids with diabetes can, and will, do anything. Done right, there truly are no boundaries.

CHAPTER 12

Support for Parents and Caregivers

Y ou've never felt more alone, yet you've never needed more support. A child's diabetes diagnosis can be an isolating experience for a parent or caregiver. Friends and neighbors who think they understand what you're going through are at times kind but misguided. Relatives sometimes back away from the hands-on support you really need. The rest of the world seems to buzz on around you, yet you can feel completely disconnected. Support from someone who truly understands can be the life vest you need, not just in the first weeks, but throughout your entire experience of raising a child with diabetes.

Why Parents Need Support

The process of accepting your child's diabetes diagnosis almost mirrors the grief process that comes with death. In a very real way, you are dealing with a loss. Your healthy, carefree child is gone, and in his place is a child who will need constant care and supervision, and about whom you will worry even more. It takes time to accept that change with grace, but it can be done.

Parents tend to react in the beginning in two distinct ways (and again, mirroring the two ways many react to a death or another crisis). They stand strong at the beginning and fall apart later on, or they collapse at the start and then regroup and become stronger. Either way, parents, for the most part, feel alone in the beginning.

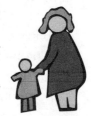

Because as much as parents would love the world to understand Type 1 and its nuances from the get-go, most parents were ignorant as well before diagnosis day. So coming home from the hospital expecting the world to be knowledgeable isn't realistic. That expectation can leave a parent feeling alienated and alone.

Bad Support

As well intentioned as it may seem, there absolutely is bad support. It comes in the form of the friend or neighbor who tells you all about her aunt who lost both legs to diabetes but still enjoyed an active knitting career, or the man in the market who reminds you that "as long as you stay away from refined sugars," your child should be fine. Bad support comes from so-called medical experts who suggest you try acupuncture instead of insulin, or who know of a special doctor who has gotten kids "off insulin for good." It's hard to stomach these lines, and many parents want to lash out, so it's a good idea to be prepared. Expect strange comments and try to remember that you once knew nothing about diabetes (even if you were smart enough to keep it to yourself).

Well Intentioned, but Not Good Support

Bad support can also come from the overzealous parent of another child with diabetes. Like militant breastfeeding mothers who insist that every mother must do the same, there are diabetes parents out there who absolutely feel their way is the only way. This can be confusing to a parent new to diabetes. They may tell you that your child's care is substandard; or that you should be working toward raising funds for a cure from day one. They may say you should not be using the insulin your doctor has told you to use. In these cases, go with your gut. Be polite and thankful, but trust your instincts with your child. If something someone says does not feel right to you, it probably isn't.

The best thing to do in these cases is to remember that these people are truly well intentioned, but that does not mean they will help you in the way you need help. Stick to your medical team's advice and ward off anything that seems questionable with a polite thank-you.

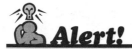

Alert!

Never accept medical advice directly from the mouths of well-intentioned friends or even other parents of kids with diabetes. Remember every child and every situation is unique. Any medical changes you consider for your child should always be run by your diabetes team first.

Good Support

Good support comes in so many forms, and in many cases, your friends will be looking for ways to help you. Good support is the parent of a child with diabetes who offers to be there for you. In this new world, nothing can better help you navigate your course than someone well into the trip.

From friends not familiar with diabetes, good support comes in the same forms it comes during any crisis. If friends ask, suggest they cook some meals that you can store, and ask them to figure out and write down the carb count per serving.

Good friends offer to attend classes to learn what diabetes is and what it means to a child's life. They know, too, that sometimes, they simply cannot do anything more than let you know they care. There is nothing more touching to a parent than the friend who truly understands what childhood diabetes is.

Finding Support

There's a wealth of support opportunities just waiting for you. Many parents don't want to reach out at first. This feeling arises partly from denial and partly from fear. Denial can be a powerful thing: "If I don't make a big deal of it, it won't be a big deal." Or, "Why would I need help? It's not like it's not a controllable disease." Fear comes for a number of reasons. Some parents fear reality, so support from parents who have lived this life means facing some realities they may not have been ready for.

Knowledgeable Support

The best thing parents and caregivers can do, though, is seek knowledgeable support. Don't worry about being forced into raising funds for one group or another; most reputable groups offering support will tell you right off that they will only help support you and that they will never suggest you donate or volunteer (more on that phase of support later in this chapter) unless that is your wish.

You'll want to find a group that offers you face-to-face support, online information, and/or a one-on-one support program that "buddies" you with other parents of children with diabetes in your area. A good combination of these options will give you a foundation for your new life with diabetes.

Meaningful Support

The first time you walk into a room full of other parents of kids with diabetes, your heart will soar, but just being in that room won't be enough. Find a support system that keeps you educated, informed, and up-to-date on diabetes care, future treatments, and cures. The one-two punch of friends who get it and an organization that keeps you on your toes will help you survive.

Look for groups that provide social time and bring in guest speakers and sales representatives from diabetes supply companies. Your support group should be your main conduit to good, up-to-date information on everything that is diabetes.

Distance Might Not Matter

While it would be nice to find support right down your block, don't hesitate to travel if you have to. Not everyone lives within a mile or two of a diabetes support group or program. If you can find one, plan ahead and make the trip. You'll realize it was worth it, even at the highest gas price. Besides, today's technology will allow you to keep in touch with those you meet there regularly, even if it isn't face-to-face.

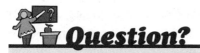

Question?

What if I'm a loner?
Online support groups may be the perfect solution for you. Just because you don't like to join groups or are not social does not mean you don't need support. Start out online and see if it leads you to more interaction.

From meetings to educational programs to online chats to Web sites, a multitude of types of support are just waiting for you. For those who entered the world of parenting a child with diabetes a decade ago, the difference in what is available is breathtaking.

Online Support

The Internet used well is a powerful and immediate tool for parents who need support, but you'll need to do more than just Google "Type 1 Diabetes." There are sites, blogs, chat rooms, and information centers that can cover every angle of diabetes, and even a few you might not want to cover.

The JDRF's Online Diabetes Support Team

For a nearly immediate response to any diabetes questions or requests for support, click on *www.jdrf.org* and hit "Online Diabetes Support Team" on their home page. The ODST is a group of nearly a hundred "Cyber Volunteers" who all do online shifts and have special areas of expertise. Say you're the parent of a toddler just diagnosed and you live in the Northwest. The ODST will connect you, via e-mail, with another parent in the Northwest whose child was diagnosed as a toddler. You'll be able to ask that person questions anonymously, and then, if you choose, they can connect you with the Juvenile Diabetes Research Foundation chapter nearest you.

The program must work. Since it's inception in 2002, the ODST has responded to more than 10,000 online support requests, and their average response time hovers at just about twenty-four hours. Some respond within an hour. Furthermore, they don't just talk to the newly diagnosed: Every age has its issues, and the ODST is there to help.

Once you've taken advantage of the ODST, they will leave it up to you if you want to reach out for in-person support or find out more about JDRF. There's no obligation, just support.

Children with Diabetes Web Site

Another great online resource is the Children with Diabetes Web site, or *www.childrenwithdiabetes.com*. This site, created by the father of a girl with diabetes, grew from a small site that parents discovered by word of mouth to one of the leaders in diabetes support. The site's parent chat room is often filled with experienced, helpful parents, and the sections of the site are like a diabetes 101 class. You can have your medical questions answered by medical experts. The site hosts special chats from time to time on subjects like holiday planning, going back to school, and dealing with teens. The site also hosts in-person conferences and events, which are discussed in the next section.

Other Web Sites

Although these two sites are the giants of online support for Type 1 diabetes and parents, there are others that offer some basics. The American Diabetes Association's Web site, *www.diabetes.org*, has a section on Type 1 and children with a lot of information, but no real-time online support is available for parents of children with Type 1. Another newer site that is growing is mychildhasdiabetes.com, which is put out by a Christian parenting group. At *www.healthatoz.com*, you can ask basic questions about Type 1 diabetes.

The best way to use the Internet is for your first outreach effort and then to keep up-to-date and in touch with other parents and on other new issues. Online support is an excellent resource that, partnered with some in-person support, can help parents feel as though they're not alone.

In-Person Support

Call it old-fashioned, but when it comes to support, the best thing is to meet with other parents who walk your walk and talk your talk. Most parents can think back to their first meeting with other parents of kids with diabetes and remember every moment and every emotion. It's a very meaningful experience, bonding with your new diabetes friends. Finding them and then finding a way to keep in touch with them will make your life and your child's life with diabetes easier to handle.

Hospital Support Groups

Some hospitals that have pediatric endocrinology departments host regular family or parent support groups. Ask your medical team if the hospital offers one, or if they know of one at a hospital or center not terribly far away. While you may not like having to travel, you will find it is well worth it. Don't hold it against your provider if they do not host a support group; many endocrine centers are understaffed and overbooked. If they are giving you good care and can point you to another place for support, stay with them and take the support where you can get it. You should also feel comfortable suggesting that your medical team hold some kind of support meeting; offer to keep it going on your own if the group seems to gel.

If you find a hospital support group that includes children, find out if you will be with your child at all times, or if you'll be breaking off into adult groups and children's groups. The best support groups give parents and caregivers a time to talk and vent well beyond little ears. Parents need a time to discuss topics, fears, and issues that shouldn't concern children at that time. If your group does include children for the entire time, expect a more upbeat, general program that kids can handle. You'll have to look for the answers to adult questions elsewhere.

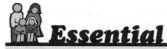 *Essential*

> When you call to inquire about a support group, ask specifically if it is for Type 1 or Type 2 diabetes, and for parents or for adults with the disease. In the beginning, particularly, you'll want to be in a room only with those who share your same situation.

Organizational Support Groups

You can find support through diabetes organizations as well. Many chapters of the Juvenile Diabetes Research Foundation hold support groups or, as some chapters call them, Parent Coffees on a monthly basis. These support groups are, for the most part, well organized and have a good history. Many Joslin Diabetes Centers host support groups as well. Go to *www.joslin.org* to find out if there is one near you. If you have the time and inclination, Children with Diabetes hosts an annual diabetes conference called "Friends for Life." Held in Orlando each July, the event is like a parents and kids diabetes summit. More information on it is available at *www .childrenwithdiabetes.com*. This organization also holds regional diabetes education sessions as well; information on these sessions is also available on their Web site.

Using Your Support

As Forrest Gump said about life, "Support is like a box of chocolates. You never know what you're going to get." In most every case with well-established groups like the JDRF, you should find a well-run program with interesting and cooperative parents. But from time to time, you might stumble across some problems. Knowing what to expect from support, how to use it, and how react to it helps parents feel good about reaching out and, in the end, makes it more worthwhile.

The Well-Meaning Parent

Let's say there's another child with diabetes in your neighborhood or school. If this is the case, chances are you're going to hear from that parent. Give her a chance, listen to what she says, and let her allow you to vent.

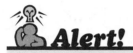

Alert!

There's a time and a place for everything and your first support experience is not a time to hear stories of gloom and doom. If you happen to stumble upon a parent with tales of woe, tell him you're not ready for that yet. If he doesn't stop, say goodbye.

The first thing parents always want to do is share diagnosis stories; your dx story will be your icebreaker until there is a cure, and hearing others' stories is somehow soothing. From there, gauge if the parent is someone you connect with: Does she seem kind enough not to push her own views on you? Was he helpful but not pushy? If they seem to be too pushy, thank them for their visit, and let them know you'll reach out to them when and if you need them. If you connect, be glad; this could be your new best friend for a while.

The Kind Stranger

If your new support comes via a support group or a connection from an organization, expect them to care about you, your child, and your current needs, not about supporting their organization. The first weeks and months are not always the best time to get involved in fundraising for a cure (see Chapter 20 for when and how to get involved). If the group or the parent focuses on your current needs and provides advice on dealing with what you are learning at this point, you've found a good thing.

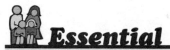

Essential

If there is no support at all for you in any of these ways, ask your school nurse to consider holding a "meet and greet" night for all parents of kids with diabetes in your town. You can take the ball and run from there.

Beware the know-it-all. This is the parent whose child always has perfect numbers and never complains. He is merely a legend in his own mind. Rather, if you can, look for a buddy or two: people you strongly connect with because of work schedules, your children's ages, or where you live. Form your own group within a group and use one another for regular support.

Becoming the Support Person

It will happen. In time, you'll find that you're ready to help others deal with diabetes and kids. It won't be in the first few weeks; it might not even be in the first year. But when the time comes, embrace that feeling and go for it. Parents everywhere need folks like you to reach out and help them. How you do it is up to you.

Pick a Program

Whether it's the JDRF's Online Diabetes Support Team or their Bag of Hope Program (see Chapter 13 for more details), a diabetes camp program, or a local hospital support group, when you're ready to help, pick the one that feels best to you. Are you better one-on-one or organizing a large group? Do you feel more empowered helping a big cause or an individual? Do you have the time to make home visits, or do you need the flexibility of helping people online and at any hour? Answering these questions will help you pinpoint which program would suit you.

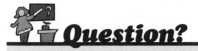 *Question?*

Will becoming the support person mean I no longer need support? Not at all; support is something parents need throughout their child's life with diabetes. Issues change, depending on the age of your child, from small kid playthings to teen issues to young adults concerns about their freedom. You'll always need help. Giving support does not mean you won't still get it.

Once you've picked a type (or types) of group that is right for you, let them know you are ready to help. Ask for training, and encourage them to be honest about your ability and where you fit. Good training should be expected of any quality outreach and support program. They owe it to you before you head out to help others.

Making It Happen on Your Own

If by chance you are in one of the few places that is too far away from any type of support, consider forming your own support group/ system. Most large organizations, like JDRF or the ADA, want to help even if they do not have a presence in your area. Contact the main support line of one of those groups and ask them to help you start a support program in your area.

In the end, reaching out, as uncomfortable as it may feel for some, is the best thing a parent can do. Imagine a world where everyone understands and knows what a high or a low is, a world where your child will never hear those odd comments. That world can, and does, exist.

CHAPTER 13

Support for Your Child

As alienated as you feel after your child's diagnosis, imagine what it does to him. Children who may have just started sleeping over at their friends' houses or earned other plums of childhood freedom now have to re-evaluate those activities along with their parents. It's even harder for teens, most of whom just want to blend with their peers. This age group struggles with feeling "different" as a norm. Finding solid support for your child, in a form he'll accept, is a priority.

Kids Need Support Even More Than You

You've felt firsthand the almost aching need for support, for a person who knows what you're going through, for a place where you feel surrounded by compatriots. As painful as that need is for you, your child probably feels it twice as much or more. From toddlers to young adults, all children need to understand that they are not the only ones who are hurting and that there are others who can share insight into this life with them. Most likely, you've sought support for yourself first, and that's okay. Think of it in terms of the oxygen mask on an airplane: In an emergency, adults are supposed to put one on their own face first and then on the child's. This isn't because you're more important; in fact, it's quite the opposite. Adults need to make themselves strong and healthy so they can care for the children around them. Now that you've found support for

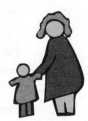

yourself and have begun feeling stronger in this new situation, it's time to focus on your child's support needs.

Tiny Tots and Support

Why would a toddler need support? The small child with diabetes may be expected to just toddle on and intellectualize later in life, but he needs to see, at the very least, that other children his age go through the same thing.

Some toddlers may be compliant from the start; others will fight finger pricks and shots. Getting them in a room or at a playground with a group of other kids their age who need to do the same thing can be a powerful message. Imagine a group of tots all frolicking in a sandbox. At the same time, the parents announce, "Okay, time to do our blood checks and have a snack." Suddenly, instead of being the only one singled out, your toddler looks around and sees *everyone* his size is doing the same thing. The subliminal message is a good one that can only help you and your child.

 Essential

While age appropriateness is vital for a support group, don't skip the idea completely if you can only find a group with older kids. Sometimes, seeing a big kid deal with diabetes has a positive impact on younger children, too.

Seeing other toddlers in action may open your little one to new ideas; a shot in a spot she's never allowed you near before, or the idea of wearing an insulin pump. While your child is still developing thoughts and feelings, it can only help to have her observe others dealing with the same issues. Savvy parents or caregivers know to find a play group that stresses kind, cooperative play and nice activities like group reading; in like manner, savvy diabetes parents find a peer group for their children with diabetes at as young an age as possible.

Tweens and Support

Tweens are perhaps the easiest group to lure into support. Still ahead of the awkward "I don't want to be with a group you force me into" stage, tweens are pretty much willing to try anything—and they need it. Preteens are usually trying to grab a bit of freedom. Whether it's giving their own shot for the first time, really considering an insulin pump (or in this day, a continuous glucose monitor), or counting the carbs in their own meals (with parental backup), tweens can learn more from each other than they ever can from either their medical team or you.

Teens and Support

This is a hard nut to crack. Teens, whether they are newly diagnosed or have been in the diabetes world for years, possibly need peer-to-peer support more than any other age group. Ironically, this is the age they most want to "blend" with their friends at school. They'll often balk at the suggestion of attending a teen diabetes group, but it's a good idea to push finding support in one way or another. After all, you can tell your teen, there are some things he is going to face that will need true insight from someone who has been there (Chapter 18 has more details on the teen years). Your teen is not going to be able to ask you about everything (in fact, he probably won't ask you at all). Tell him that if he has the support and input of other teens with diabetes, you'll be more comfortable giving him more freedom in life.

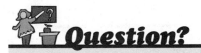

Question?

Is "group attendance bribery" okay?
Bribery isn't the best strategy in parenting, but bargaining can be. Try for example, "If you attend this group regularly, I won't be as worried about you going boating all day long." That way the child sees an inherent reward in attending the group.

Teens need a place where they can talk, safely, about issues they just may not be able to discuss with you. It's hard to swallow, but it's part of life. The parent who helps her teen find the place to work that out ends up better off.

Where to Find Help

It would be nice if diabetes support groups for all ages were as ubiquitous as, say, Dunkin' Donuts or Waffle Houses, but alas, they are not. Finding a group at all can be a challenge. Finding one that fits your child's needs perfectly can be even more difficult. But with creativity, footwork, and a bit of luck, you can make it happen.

Through Your Health-Care Provider

If only every pediatric endocrinology program came with built-in support groups; unfortunately, this is not always the case. Your first step in looking for a group should be talking with your medical team, most likely with the social worker. Oftentimes, even if programs don't have support groups, they do have special seasonal events like Halloween parties or holiday events. Sometimes, tapping into these can be a great first step toward finding good support groups. In fact, if you have older children, suggesting they volunteer for events like this geared at smaller children can be a great way to open the door to some supportive relationships.

 Essential

One-on-one support can be great for kids, too. Ask your medical team if they would consider "matching" your child and family with another one in your area, so you can find a peer with the same background for your child.

Your team should also know which groups offer support for kids. Remember, it does not have to be a group of patients all from the same center. Kids with diabetes are kids with diabetes, and they can bond no matter where they are cared for. Some parents of older kids report that having their child serve as a "role model" to a younger child helped their teen become more outgoing about good diabetes care. And conversely, caregivers of little ones say they love having a "big diabetes friend" to look up to. Your medical team might be able to help you make such relationships happen.

Through Organizations

Many organizations, both local and nationally based, have family and child support programs. The Juvenile Diabetes Research Foundation has more than eighty chapters across the country. Although some rural families may not find one near them, most people who live close to cities or in well-populated suburbs can find help.

 Essential

The JDRF's Bag of Hope program is a great way for your child to get her first taste of support. A local family comes to your home with a bag of goodies, including a teddy bear with diabetes. Go to ✑*www .jdrf.org* for more details.

The American Diabetes Association holds many educational forums and special events throughout the year. You may be able to find good spots for your children to meet other children at these events.

The Children with Diabetes Foundation hosts the annual Friends for Life Conference each July in Orlando, as well as regional conferences across the country all year long. Some local hospitals and groups offer programs for families as well. Finding them could be as simple as asking your school nurse, who should be up-to-date on such programs.

Diabetes Camps

The natural place for your child to find support is at a diabetes camp. Once limited in numbers, camps seem to be everywhere now. While some older kids may be resistant to a diabetes camp experience, it's in their best interest that you push them to give it a try. A week, or more, spent in a place where everyone understands, everyone is on board, and everyone has to do the same things can be more than therapeutic to a child; it can be life-changing.

How Long and at What Age

For the most part, children need to be eight or older to attend the overnight programs, but there are exceptions. Some "mini camps" last just a few nights and take younger children. Others will consider taking younger children after meeting them and seeing they are capable of the experience. How do you know if your child is ready? A simple first step is to talk to him and then talk to the camp about him.

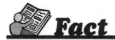 **Fact**

A great resource for finding a diabetes camp in your area is the Diabetes Education and Camping Association's Web site, *www .diabetescamps.org*. There you can find listings by state and even by country.

For children who have a diabetes buddy, camp may be an easier sell. Even if your child doesn't have a friend to go with, show him the camp's Web site and he'll see that all the children have fun there. Point out that the camp isn't a week-long lesson on diabetes; rather, it is a classic camp that intertwines life with diabetes with life as a regular camping kid.

While younger children (say, nine and under) may want to opt for a shorter camp time, most kids want at least two full weeks. Camp programs tend to run through a session-long agenda, and children who leave early will feel as if they are missing something. If you do decide to send your child, try at least a full two-week session. They'll thank you for it. For younger children who are not ready, consider day camp. It's just as good but without the sleepovers.

What Makes a Good Camp?

A good camp has a background of helping kids with diabetes. A good camp has medical staff on-site, including nurses in almost every cabin and an endocrinologist on-site at all times. Alumni participation is a definite sign of a good camp; warm feelings that last a lifetime usually mean something special is going on.

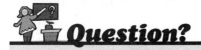 *Question?*

Will my child outgrow camp?
Not if you encourage her to work as a counselor. Diabetes camp counseling is a win-win-win situation. Your child is in a safe environment, has a steady summer job, and is being a role model for younger kids with diabetes.

Good camps have lots of regular camp activities and are not right out front with diabetes education. Put aside your visualization of your child sitting in a classroom with a lecturer pointing at a diagram of a pancreas. Good camps blend it all: like the camp play that spoofs *The Wizard of Oz* where Dorothy is attacked by extra carbs instead of monkeys; or the craft activity where kids invent and draw the "most amazing pump ever."

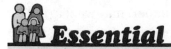 **Essential**

> Ask any camp you are considering for a sample weekly activity schedule. It will give you a glimpse into how they do things, what types of activities they stress, and the importance they placed on certain diabetic concerns.

Without a doubt, the best thing that good camps do is gather kids so they have time just to talk. Campers repeatedly tell their parents that while they love their family and home, their camp friends are the only people who truly understand. That's because they're tucked away in a cabin with their true and complete peers: a group of same-age kids who are battling the same disease. It's a powerful experience.

Parental Involvement During Camp

Most good camps will ask parents from the start if they want to be called every time a dose change is considered, or if they want to leave it up to the camp's medical staff. Here's a suggestion (and this is a personal decision): Leave it up to the camp staff. One of the beautiful things about camp is that it gives parents and caregivers, who are now 24/7 medical caretakers, time off. Caring for a child with diabetes can be all-consuming and exhausting, and it comes with burnout. Letting the camp take control for a couple of weeks can be just the boost you need to face the next year of care.

In addition, there are so many changes at camp. Kids go nonstop. They are often hot. Most kids need way less insulin at camp than at home, so being called constantly about these kinds of questions without being able to be there might provide even more stress. If your camp is staffed with medical professionals and most of the counselors have diabetes themselves, consider taking a break. You'll find you look forward to it each year.

Online Support

When it comes to kids and online support, parents need to be careful. Online communication is a natural for our kids, much more so than it was or ever will be for those of us who grew up before the 1990s. Before you let your child take part in online support for kids, make sure you check out the site for authenticity and safety. Once you find a few good sites and you know you can monitor them, online support can work great for kids who need to talk to others in their situation.

Chat Rooms

By now, most astute parents know that any chat room you let your child enter simply must be checked out by you first. Find out if there is a capable adult administrator, if they are backed up or supported by a known organization, if there are set topics, and how moderating the site works.

One quality spot for teens with diabetes to chat not just for support but for education is Diabetes Teen Talk (*www.diabetesteentalk.com*). Started by well-known youth diabetes advocate Allison Blass, the site has useful information, interesting polls, and regular chats that draw in world experts on diabetes and teens. The site even has a section that enables you to get to know the teens who run it and find out all about them.

Children with Diabetes also has a teen chat site, and since you can chat at the parents' site at the same time, you can check in on your child and "see" what he is chatting about at all times. CWD has a large group of moderators who take shifts online and who instantly kick out anyone who is chatting inappropriately.

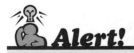

Alert!

Be wary of temporary chats set up on general message boards. Most are not moderated and can include people you don't want your child chatting with. In other words, only trust a well-established online site.

Your child's camp may set up winter chats as well, inviting campers who were at her session to "reunite" online to catch up on life, talk camp, and lend some between-session support. If your camp is not doing this, you may want to suggest it.

Other Online Choices

Kids know all kind of online meeting spots now: Xanga, MySpace. com, Facebook. While in theory, they are all excellent ways for kids to communicate around the world, you need to keep close tabs on them. If you allow your child to have such a site and join a diabetes group in it, insist that he keeps his site "private" and even then, make a weekly check of whom he has added as "allowed friends." Unless he can give you a connection you know is real, remove any questionable "friends" when you discover them.

Some sites have "passive interaction" with information, stories, and feedback options but no live chats. JDRF Kids online (*kids.jdrf .org*) is one such site. These sites are like an online magazine, giving kids insight into feelings, ideas, and even some celebrities who share their challenges.

The American Diabetes Association has a youth zone on their Web site (*www.diabetes.org*, click on Youth Zone) that offers kids basics in diabetes information, games, and even a kid kit they can get for free. There is also a teen message board that your child can use to post questions and receive answers.

Used well, online chats and sites can make kids feel part of a community. In a world where most kids with diabetes are the only one in their school, a place online where they are one of many can be most welcome.

Publications

Everyone in America wants to feel as if there's a publication just for them. There's even a magazine for snowman collectors. So of course, kids with diabetes want their own magazines and books as well. The good news is they are out there.

Magazines

Countdown for Kids, a publication tucked into each issue of the JDRF's *Countdown* magazine, features topics that kids care about, like burnout or lying to parents, and presents them in a way that's fun and easy to digest. Their running comic series about Pump Boy (and his good friend Hot Shot) is popular among kids and even some parents. Their simple discussions on science and research explain diabetes issues so clearly that many adults read them for a more accessible explanation of science topics, as for example, the story explaining islet cells starring Sally the Cell.

Diabetes Forecast, published by the American Diabetes Association, also has a kid's section in each issue that discusses things in more understandable terms.

Books

For younger kids, the workbook *It's Time to Learn about Diabetes* is a fun, interactive way to embrace what they need to know about their disease. The large pages are crayon friendly and really do explain things in a simple way. Look for the angry ketone!

Also for younger kids, *I'm Tougher than Diabetes* tells the story of life with diabetes through the words and photos of real kids.

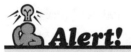

Alert!

Writing can be therapeutic. Encourage your child, no matter her age, to put her diabetes story on paper. Toddlers can draw; teens can journal. It's all a great way to get things out in the open, and in the future your child can look back at her writing and be inspired by all that she has been through.

For older kids, *Sugar Was My Best Food* was written by a young teen with Type 1 and addresses issues from his point of view. It's a bit dated because pumps were not readily available when it was published, but it rings true all the same.

One warning when it comes to older teen books such as *Needles*, a memoir about life with diabetes. Read them first, and make sure you want your child exposed to what is in there.

When Basic Support Isn't Enough

You've reached out for support for your child, both in groups and online and still, something isn't right. Your child is struggling and feels alone. She seems moody and starts to resent diabetes. It may be time to seek expert help.

Taking the Step

If you suspect your child may be suffering from depression or struggling more than you would expect a child with diabetes to struggle, it's time to get help. Your first step should be to talk to your endocrinologist and social worker. They may arrange an immediate meeting with your child to assess the situation. Tell them beforehand all your concerns. Be specific about actions, words, or events that concerned you. Then, expect your medical team to talk more to your child than to you. They may want to talk to him alone, and this is a good thing. As much as you love your child, he may feel more comfortable talking without you there.

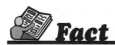 **Fact**

> Don't feel alone. Many children with diabetes, particularly teens, struggle at some point and need some kind of therapeutic help. This is a chance to help your child be happier in life and know that most other kids fight these battles, too.

Your team can assess whether they feel your child needs to meet with the social worker more often, or with a therapist near home on a regular basis, or just continue to cope with things. If they tell you things are fine and you still feel doubtful, go with your instincts. As always, it's safer to err on the side of caution.

How to Get the Right Therapist

Unfortunately, you cannot just open the phone book and find a child therapist who specializes in diabetes issues. If you are lucky, your medical team (particularly the social worker) will know someone in your area who has good experience treating a child with diabetes. If not, you're going to have to do some hunting. Do not be afraid to quiz the therapists on diabetes. If they know little and admit it, that's okay, as long as they are willing to listen and learn. If they think they know diabetes and really only understand Type 2, you may want to keep on looking.

Most of all trust your child's reaction to the person. Your child must give it more than one chance, but if, after three or more sessions, your child does not feel a connection, trust her (and show her you respect her feelings), and move on to another therapist. In the end, a good therapist can help a child adjust not just to life with diabetes but to life in general—and that is a bonus.

Most parents and caregivers find that recognizing their child's need for real support and being proactive about it helps keep them ahead of trouble. Wise parents do just that.

CHAPTER 14

The Honeymoon Period

I t doesn't happen to everyone, but for those who experience it, the "honeymoon period" in a child's diabetes can be a sigh of relief. During this period, the child's pancreas is still producing a relatively good amount of insulin and her blood sugars are easier to handle. For parents, it can be a time to learn, adapt to diabetes, and sometimes, slip into denial. This time is a double-edged sword.

What Is the Honeymoon Period?

For some children, particularly those whose diabetes is diagnosed earlier in the beta cell–destruction process, there is a honeymoon period. During this time, the child's insulin-producing cells in the pancreas are still working at some level. It is thought that the autoimmunity that is determined to destroy most—if not all—of your child's insulin-producing cells has not yet completed its job, and those cells still functioning can even step it up a bit, desperately trying to make up for the destroyed cells.

For children, this can mean easy-to-control blood sugars. For parents, it can mean less stress since they may not see a lot of highs and may find that tiny bits of insulin do the trick.

"Remission" or Not?

Some people like to call the honeymoon period a "remission" from diabetes. This can be a tricky term. First of all, there truly is no remission from the autoimmunity that causes Type 1 diabetes. Once your child's body has flipped that switch for whatever reason (see Chapter 1 for a discussion on what causes Type 1 diabetes), there is no flipping it back or even putting it on hold. Calling this period a remission can send some dangerous suggestions to the minds of a child and a parent.

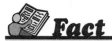 ***Fact***

> While there is no true test to confirm that a child is in a honeymoon period, endocrinologists tend to think that a child who maintains an A1c of about 6.5 or lower with little insulin or effort is in a honeymoon period.

The term *remission* can also send the wrong message to friends, family, and other concerned people. One of the most frustrating things about living with diabetes is the inability to change the path of the disease, coupled with the public perception that once you get things "under control" or "regulated" with a healthy diet and good medical plan, it's a snap. This is simply not the case. As hard as it is to come to terms with—and take a deep breath here, because this isn't easy to accept—there will be no remission for your child. However, although no honeymoon lasts forever, it's perfectly okay to embrace and enjoy the good that comes with any time in life.

Identifying the Honeymoon

Once you get past the initial shock and often crisis of diagnosis, you brace yourself for constantly changing insulin doses and somewhat frightening numbers on your child's meter screen. You take a deep breath and then—it's almost a snap. Diabetes may not be a big deal after all. If a short time after diagnosis, you begin to notice that things are relatively easy to handle, your child is in a honeymoon period.

Children in these periods often require tiny amounts of insulin; sometimes as close to none as you can imagine. Parents and caregivers well into their diabetes experience with their child look back and laugh at learning to have the hand-eye coordination to be able to draw up a quarter-unit of insulin for a child. They smile, too, at the time when a blood sugar of 200 sent them into a panic. All these events are signs of a honeymoon.

Another sign can be seen right in your logbooks. If you're tracking numbers (and you should be) and you can count your child's highs for a week on one hand, your child is in a honeymoon.

One test that can help let you know if your child is honeymooning is the C-peptide test. C-peptides decrease as her ability to produce insulin decreases. A child without diabetes usually comes in at about 1.5. Once a child is 0.8 or lower, the honeymoon is over. Most endocrinologists don't think the test is warranted. A honeymoon is so recognizable that most physicians can tell you just from your reports if your child is experiencing one.

 Essential

Diluted insulin can be a great choice during a honeymoon period. If you find you're drawing up doses so tiny you can barely see them, talk to your team about diluting insulin. It can make your life easier, and done right is perfectly acceptable.

How to Cope

Although the term *honeymoon* provides warm and fuzzy feelings, coping can be a challenge for parents and children. In other words, it may be a honeymoon, but it's not all hearts, roses, and target-range blood sugars.

Your Perception (the Good)

When you think of how few people truly understand the basics of Type 1 diabetes, never mind the intricacies, you realize, quickly, that almost no one out there understands what a honeymoon is and what it means. This can lead to some skewed perceptions of life with Type 1, of its impact on your child, and of your ability (or inability) to manage the disease.

For you, the shock of leaving the hospital and the fear of mastering this complicated new life can be immediately quelled by a nice honeymoon—and there's nothing wrong with embracing that. Think of it this way: If you were asked to run a marathon with only four days to train, you'd have a heck of a time even crossing the finish line, never mind winning. But given a full year (or more) to get the feel for the run and to work your way up to the real run, you might just do okay. A honeymoon can be the same for parents.

The Downside

This is one honeymoon that is not all hearts and roses. Putting aside the fact that you and your child are struggling emotionally to accept a chronic disease, and that you are feeling alienated and afraid, the physical aspects of honeymooning can be tricky. Although it's a good thing for the body to produce its own insulin for as long as possible, it's also a complicated thing.

 Essential

Blood glucose testing is more important than ever during the honeymoon, since lows are a possibility. Stick to the times and plan that your team suggests. Letting your testing slack off can endanger your child's health. Be diligent.

During the honeymoon, your child's body produces insulin in sporadic doses. Unlike the body of a child without diabetes, you cannot predict exactly what the pancreas is going to do each time your child eats or plays or sleeps or just lives. Toss a shot or bolus of added insulin into this, and you can have some dicey times.

That's why lows are a big concern during the honeymoon. Most medical teams help families err on the side of caution, giving lower doses and expecting to correct for a high from time to time. Some parents get so frustrated with their inability to judge what the child's insulin needs will be that they actually express relief when the honeymoon is over, and it's all down to the insulin you personally place into your child's body.

Your Child's Perception (the Good)

A good honeymoon can help a child have time to adapt as well. It's not easy, for a child of any age, to grasp and accept all that comes with diabetes graciously, maturely, and without complaint. A honeymoon period can mean fewer shots and certainly a longer period to begin to understand the feelings that come physically with highs and lows, and emotionally with being a child with "something different."

The child who experiences a long honeymoon will get some breathing space and be able to see that he can live with diabetes. By not diving directly into the period when blood sugars can bounce quickly high or low with a confused carb count or a miscalculated insulin dose, he can see that diabetes is not always a reason for panic. Finally, by experiencing a high here and there and from time to time rather than often, he can get used to the concept of going a little high sometimes without panic.

Public Perception

By now you realize that most of the world thinks that if you just keep your child away from jelly doughnuts, you should be fine. The impact of diabetes on a child (and a family's) life is widely misunderstood. A honeymoon, as great as it is, can feed into those misguided perceptions. When your child's blood sugars fall into line with relative ease, friends and family may think that indeed diabetes is no big deal. Naysayers may be convinced that diabetes is not a disease that must be cured. You'll need to find a way to explain the honeymoon period to your friends and family without them chiding you for being so pessimistic and suggesting that perhaps your child won't develop full diabetes.

Encourage your friends to investigate the Type 1 honeymoon period. Entering that term into a search engine will bring up a wealth of information that should quell their comments that long bike rides and low carbs will prevent high blood sugar in your child.

Hope and Denial

Get ready, because if your child is in a honeymoon, you're going to wonder if there was a mistake in your child's diagnosis. As wonderful as a honeymoon can be, it can also trick the best of minds. Hope and denial are powerful emotions. Keeping them in check during this time is important to long-term emotional well-being.

Your Own Wishes

What parent would not hope the doctors were wrong? No one can easily accept that their perfect child has an incurable disease that means a daily, sometimes hourly, struggle. A honeymoon, more often than not, leaves a parent doubting her team's diagnosis.

So what's a parent to do? First and foremost, go ahead and ask your medical team. Don't worry about insulting them; they are used to being asked this very question. Let them explain why they are certain their diagnosis is correct. Don't listen to any outsiders; urban legends of diabetes just going away abound. You need to trust your team. If you still cannot let go of that doubt, ask your primary care physician to get you a second, independent opinion.

Your Arrogance

This can also be a time when caregivers assume their child's good numbers are simply because they are better at diabetes care than anyone else. First of all, you *are* great at caring for your child. The fact that you take the time to read books and learn all you can about care means you're a champion for your child. Second, that does not mean the reason his numbers are within target now is just you. There will come a time when the honeymoon ends, and you'll still be that amazing parent. Do not assign your self-worth as a parent to blood sugars. Rather, assign it to the effort and love you put into the situation, no matter the short-term outcomes.

Your Child's Wishes

No wish can be stronger (or more expected to become reality) than that of a child. With very small children, the idea of diabetes in general will be an unwelcome one, and even in a honeymoon period, your child is adapting to what they see, in their small-child mind (and rightfully so), as a major life adjustment. For the smaller child, a shot is a shot and a finger poke is a finger poke. More predictable numbers or less need to adjust doses is not going to affect their point of view.

But an older child—and that is any child who can reason or understand expectations—can be tricked by a honeymoon period. Your child may notice that the high blood sugar feeling that was so acute at diagnosis time really has not come around again. She may find that it's easy to know what dose she needs for certain foods or activities. Encourage her to enjoy this rather peaceful diabetes time, but make sure you say it out loud: "Your diabetes is not going away."

A Time to Learn and Explore

If your child is in a honeymoon period, don't just rest on the realization that you've got a little time to chill. Use this time to learn, explore, and try out all the things you need to understand to make life normal for your child.

Trial Runs

Houston conducts trial runs all the time for space shuttle lift-offs; now you can do it for your child and all the things he wants to do in life. A trial run of all sorts of special events, from a birthday party to a beach day, will help you figure out the basics of handling such events before you actually have to do them. In other words, here is your chance to screw up in private so you can get it right later.

Say your child is a big lacrosse player and you're dreading the start of the season. How will play affect her blood sugar? What kind of snacks should you use during the game? During this honeymoon period, gather a group of her favorite friends and players and hold a mock-game in your backyard or at a local park. Make it as long as a real game is; make sure your child plays as much as she usually will, and check her blood sugars more times than you can imagine. Play with things like watered-down energy drinks and granola bars, and see what works best. Although things will change once the honeymoon is over, the basics will stay the same.

Product Trials

The honeymoon is a great time, too, to discuss new products and therapies with your medical team. (See Chapter 6 for details on what's out there now.) Sometimes, long-acting insulin or a pump, used well, can be a great way to extend a honeymoon. At the very least, this time of less erratic blood sugars is a great time to check out some other options and give them a try (always, *always* under the direct supervision of your medical team).

Your team may say you are too new to diabetes to try options other than what they have initially suggested. While in the end it is best to follow their expert advice, don't be afraid to push your suggestions a bit. Go into your appointments armed with knowledge. If you understand what changing to a longer-acting insulin and more short-acting boluses means, your team is more likely to consider helping you try something new. If you head in knowing all about pumps, they'll understand that you want to try something else and are willing to learn all you need to make it happen.

Can the Honeymoon Be Extended?

Who doesn't want a honeymoon to last forever? The diabetes honeymoon is no exception. Patients and doctors have long struggled with finding a way to make the honeymoon last. Although there is nothing concrete yet, progress is being made.

Why Longer Is Better

It's not just about your mental health, your child's mental health, and giving you all space and time to adapt to life with diabetes, although arguably, those are good enough reasons to extend a honeymoon. A long honeymoon means that your child's blood sugar average and A1c is closer to the target range for a longer period. Put simply, lower A1cs mean less damage to the body. Many studies have shown that tighter control over a long time lessens the impact that diabetes can have on the body, particularly the extremities and internal organs.

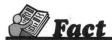 **Fact**

The daddy of all complications and control studies is the Diabetes Control and Complications Trial. The trial took place from 1983 to 1993 and changed the way Type 1 diabetes is treated. For details, go to ✐*http://diabetes.niddk.nih.gov/dm/pubs/control/.*

In addition, a long honeymoon means the islet cells that are still producing insulin may be able to last longer and not work as hard. The longer your child's body can produce its own insulin, the better off he is. Not only will he need less injected insulin, but he could hold on to insulin-producing cells for a time, in the future, when scientists may know how to help those cells regenerate (see Chapter 21 for potential cures).

How to Extend the Honeymoon

Follow the plan your diabetes team builds with you for your child. While it may seem like a nice goal not to have to give insulin at all, most experts agree that some amount of insulin, even the tiniest bit, is good for your child. This is because you don't want the remaining cells to overwork themselves and die too quickly, and because your child's body absolutely needs to have enough insulin at all times. Honeymoons can be tricky: the body can work in bursts and breaks, and sometimes, you'll have no idea what that pancreas is doing or thinking. With an insulin plan, you'll at least make sure that your child's body always has insulin of some kind in it, avoiding major highs and diabetic ketoacidosis.

Extending the Honeymoon

Scientists and researchers are working to find a way to extend the honeymoon. In fact, most newly diagnosed patients are now being told about a few studies that are trying to stop the progression of the destruction of the insulin-producing cells. Discuss this possibility with your medical team. If you're interested, ask them to guide you to good studies. A list of the studies, what they entail, and who can be part of them is available at *www.diabetestrialnet.org*.

Make sure you consider all the ramifications of a study, including time constraints, center locations, possible side effects, and most important, how your child feels about taking part in it. In the end, even if it sounds like your dream come true, remember it's your child's body and he should have a say. He's already dealing with enough. So, if he wants a study, great; if not, keep his wishes in mind.

When It's Over

It's going to happen. It might happen quickly, but more often it's a slow realization: The diabetes honeymoon is over. How long it takes to get to that point is part chance, but how you react to it is all skill. Handling this time with both emotional and technical skills is a challenge, but one you must face.

Timing

Honeymoons can last from a month to as long as a year and a half. Some doctors claim to have seen rare cases that lasted as long as three years. One Boston physician tells of a patient whose honeymoon lasted a full six years. On average, though, if your child experiences a honeymoon, expect it to last from six months to a year at best.

As time goes by and you settle in, you'll begin to notice more spikes in blood sugars and/or a need for more insulin to cover carbs. You'll look at your week's logbook and begin to see trends. Usually lunch and dinner are the first times to show spikes in blood sugars, but each child is different. As you see these trends and talk to your team about upping doses, the realization will begin to set in for you, your child, and your team that the honeymoon is ending.

Timing of the honeymoon's end can sometimes be complicated by timing in life. For instance, most children's insulin needs go up when school starts (there is more downtime and less outdoor frolicking). You may think that the honeymoon is ending when it's actually just a normal life-adjustment time that you'll come to expect every year.

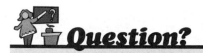

Question?

Is it important to pinpoint a time when the honeymoon ends?
Not really. In fact, it might be less emotional for your child if you just quietly transition into the nonhoneymoon time. This way it will be one less thing for you and your child to mourn.

Parents can see why, during the honeymoon and just after, it is particularly important to be meticulous about keeping records. The only way you and your team are going to be able to make smart decisions on dose changes will be by studying your logbooks. Keep them and keep them well, so that the transition can go relatively well for your child's physical well-being.

Accepting the End

Parents and caregivers, even more than children, have a hard time accepting the end of the honeymoon and the beginning of the rest of diabetes. First, parents who were sure they could master diabetes to the point of practically nondiabetic averages find out that in fact, nature can be a bear when it comes to blood sugars. If you feel let down, talk to someone, either in your support group or on your health team. She'll tell you that you are not alone; more than one parent has been fooled by a nice honeymoon. She'll also remind you of how well you used that honeymoon time and how much you've learned.

It can also be difficult to accept that you're going to have to deal with some erratic blood sugars from time to time. Soon, gone will be the days when your heart nearly stops at a 300. Yes, you'll still react quickly and treat it as it should be treated, but in the end, you'll remember that diabetes is a marathon, not a sprint. Some miles you're going to stall a bit on; others you'll fly through. Honeymoon or not, it's all about the finish line. With your child, you are doing all you can to find the pace that makes the run a pleasant and healthful one for both of you.

CHAPTER 15

Independence and What It Means

No matter your child's age, the diabetes diagnosis means taking a step backward in independence and reworking how you'll let your child "go." Finding ways to allow children to feel independent is an important challenge and a giant step toward showing your child how to live a new normal life. This chapter will cover independence that is age-appropriate for your child, what to do in situations that demand your child's independence, and how to give your child the skills to take control of her life.

Age-Appropriate Independence

As is the case in raising children in general, there are age-appropriate levels of independence. Parents need to find a way to walk a fine line between making sure their child is safe and not hovering over them or holding them back.

Little Ones

For smaller children with diabetes, independence only becomes an issue as they begin to notice other children go play at a friend's house without their parents along. At the preschool and even early elementary age, this is not easy to do and, frankly, cannot be done without parents of friends who are willing to learn about your child's diabetes needs.

Usually, a first big step for little ones is the ability to do their own finger prick and even shot. That event calls for a celebration. Proud parents call relatives and friends and even give their child a congratulatory gift. But there's no need to celebrate too much. The longer you control your child's care, the more you'll push back burnout.

 Essential

If your small child wants to change her pump sites or give herself shots or prick her fingers, find a way to still be part of it. A child this age is in no way ready to handle this medical responsibility completely on her own.

When your child can do these tasks and a friend is willing to learn about diabetes, it's probably okay to let your child begin play dates without you there. But you'll still need to check in if the playtime is longer than two hours. Agree with the other parent that you'll call in two hours, and let them know ahead of time what you'll need to know: your child's blood sugar and what he's eaten since arriving. By checking in quietly, your child can play independently but still have your watchful eye on him, making sure all is fine.

School-Age Children

By second or third grade, children begin to want to do things without their parents holding their hand. Whether it's a bike ride around their cul-de-sac, a birthday party, or a movie night with another family, your child will want to head out without you by this point, and that can be hard for a parent.

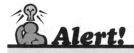

Alert!

By the time your child is school-age, you need to let go a tiny bit as a parent. If you find you simply cannot, it's time to sit down with your medical team and get to the bottom of your feelings. In order for your child to live a somewhat normal life, you'll need to give him some independence at this age.

Since children this age understand numbers, and children who have had diabetes for a number of years even know their goal range, it's okay, with the advent of the cell phone, to come up with a plan for your child to participate in these activities. But be aware, this will take planning and discussion. You and your child will need to figure out how to make it work and even go on a test run, in which your child acts out how the event will take place without you there. Your first step will be to set a schedule and write it down. Explain to your child that you'll need to share this with the supervising adult, if it's a movie night or birthday party. If we're talking about a bike ride around the block, encourage your child to set the alarm on his wristwatch to remind him that it's time to head home and check in, or at least call.

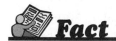

Fact

Kids who have diabetes supply bags tend to forget less. Find a cute bag that your daughter does not mind carrying and keep it ready for outings by filling it with strips, an extra meter, and carbs.

Once you've set the plan and discussed it with your child, talk to the parent in charge and let him know that while you are working toward some kind of independence, your child should never be completely on his own. If the parent cannot agree to remind your child of a schedule and watch as your child checks levels, boluses, or takes a shot, then you need to say no. Sometimes, other parents will act in ways that you know are not safe for your child, such as not following your orders. If this happens, explain to your child that it is better if his friend comes to play at your house instead.

The Slumber Party

First off, it's safe to say that all parents, not just those of kids with diabetes, dread the age of slumber parties. Nowadays, parents seem to be pushing them at younger and younger ages. You, however, need to base your decision on more than just age.

If You Feel the Time Is Right

So your child has asked enough times and the child who's hosting the party has a trustful parent. You've decided to leap into the world of sleepovers. You'll need to come up with a masterful plan that, whether your child likes it or not, will include you checking in.

First, plan to have your child check her blood sugars every two hours the entire time she is awake. This can be tricky, since kids tend to stay up very late for sleepovers. But the reality is, with the excitement and the energy burned, your child will need to keep a close eye on blood sugars, and the parent in charge will need to assist you in this. Set a target range that is a little higher than usual, and let your child and the parent know that as long as your child is in that range, he doesn't need to call you. But if your child goes low or extremely high, he'll need to call, no matter what the hour.

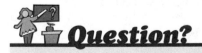 **Question?**

How much higher should I run my child for sleepovers?
A safe amount is about 30 points higher than their usual target range, with extra carbs at bedtime if they are 130 or lower. Better to err a bit higher on these nights than be sorry later.

If you find that your child is extra high or low at bedtime, you'll need to talk to the parent and find out if he wants to do a middle-of-the-night blood check or if he'd rather you come over to do it. Let him know it's just to be safe, and you are almost sure things will be fine. Yet, with the added activity and food, it has to be done.

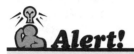

Alert!

Be wary of junk foods at slumber parties, not because your child cannot have them, but because bowls of snacks are everywhere, and it can be hard to keep track of what your child has eaten. Insist that she count out chips or candies ahead of time into her own bowl so she knows what to bolus and eat.

You'll also need to let the parents and your child know that you expect them to check right after she wakes up in the morning and to call you to check in. Kids forget or use this event as a chance to escape their routine. But a morning check is crucial in this situation.

If the Time Feels Wrong

As stated at the start of this section, even parents and caregivers of kids without diabetes aren't big fans of sleepovers. Children often eat poorly and sleep poorly. They can come home cranky and exhausted, spent for the entire next day, and all of that can mess with blood sugars.

So what if you'd just like to say no? Your child will argue that you're treating him differently; that you're letting diabetes rule his life. And in some ways, you are. It depends on what your issues are.

If it is a case of not trusting other parents to follow your requests, you can still have your child take part in slumber parties. But here's the hook: They'll *all* have to be at your house. Some parents who aren't comfortable with their children sleeping over other homes have made that deal: As long as it would be a time you'd otherwise say yes, you'll always allow it to be at your house. The bonus to that situation is all the other parents in town will idolize you for taking the party out of their home and putting it in yours.

If you just don't feel your child is ready, then as long as you have the same rule for all your other children, it's fine. If your child has not been responsible or smart about her care recently, it's okay to keep her home. It's not a punishment; it's a safety issue. Explain to your child that because she's lied or skipped checks, you are not ready to trust her away from you. Give her a goal: one week of not skipping and she can go back to a party again. Remember, you have to stick to what you say.

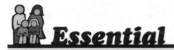

Essential

The great thing about hosting a slumber party is that you control the food portions, monitor the sleeping time (to a point), and keep a close eye on your child throughout the event. The downside is you'll have a slumber party and many overexcited children at your house.

High School Freedom

High school is the time your child will want to take the most personal control of his diabetes. Parents need to be careful how much they let or don't let this happen. Your teen is laying the groundwork for independence, but it needs to be done slowly.

School Responsibilities

Teens won't want to check in with you or their nurse in high school, yet you'll need to find a way to keep track of what is going on in their lives. It's a good idea to schedule an endocrinologist or CDE appointment in the late summer before each school year. Let the expert help you lay down a plan with your high school student. There should be set times each day when your child must check, and there should be a way for you to make sure he has at the end of each school day.

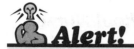

Alert!

Do not use multiple meters during the high school years. You'll want to have all the data in one meter, and not give your child an excuse such as, "Oh, I was 104. It's at school on my other meter." Keep all the information together.

If your teen is involved in sports, you may want to ask her to give you a call before any away game you are not attending. A quick check-in to talk about how her day has gone and how to deal with the sporting event can help. She won't like this, but you need to push your support on her when she wants to be independent.

Parties, Dances, and Dates

So, what about events like the prom and homecoming that keep them out all night? You don't want to deny your child these rites of passage, but you need to make sure he is safe. Know the dates well ahead of time, and remind your teen that he'll need to prove his trustworthiness well before that event comes. He must show that he is mature enough to be trusted for an entire night of parties. If he fails to earn your trust, consider holding the after-party at your house. Yes, you'll have a sleepless night, but you'd probably be worried anyway.

As discussed in Chapter 18, you'll need to encourage your teen to be honest about alcohol and drugs. Combined with diabetes, they are dangerous at best, and if your child betrays your trust and ends up in a dire situation, you'll need to be the responsible parent and not allow her another opportunity. Cigarettes, too, are a must-avoid for people with diabetes, because they dramatically increase the rate of major diabetic complications. Hard as it is, sometimes independence is the opposite of what a high school student truly needs.

She'll think her life is over if you deny her a party, but you'll know it's for her long-term safety and health.

When to Say Goodbye to the School Nurse

She's been your best ally for years now, and you hate to think how you'll get by without her. But there will come a time your child wants to spend less time at the nurse's office and more time in the class-room. Transitioning to this form of independence takes care as well.

How to Know the Timing Is Right

If your child has had diabetes for a few years and has proven her ability to master finger pokes and boluses, you can consider her request for independence at school. Often this issue arises when a child is transitioning into a new grade or even a new school. The child believes he's mature enough to be able to handle things in the classroom and may not have the same thrill of going to the nurse as he did as a smaller child, when it was cool to pick a friend to bring along.

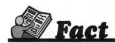 **Fact**

Every school district has its own rules. Check with yours about whether it allows children to carry their own diabetes supplies. If it does not, have a meeting and request that the district change that rule. Be prepared for your meeting with statistics and facts on your child's need for independent care; a well-thought-out argument may be your best advocate in changing a district's established rules.

Middle school and high school are prime times for kids to want to make this change. If you think your child is ready, you'll need to do a few things. First, come up with a plan that you can actually see your child is following. Second, ask your child to see the nurse for at least the first week of school, so she builds some kind of a relationship with this new nurse.

Your child will need to understand that this independence comes with responsibilities, and you'll be checking that she is sticking to them. Let her know that if she deviates from the plan, you'll ask her to go back to the nurse again for a time. Independence in this case is a privilege not a right.

Back to the Original Plan

So what if you start out with your child free from the nurse and it does not seem to work? Parents should never hesitate to take a step back in care and independence. Before you start the new plan, however, make sure you outline your expectations and the possible repercussions to your child. Have him repeat them back to you; consider putting them in writing. Be as clear as you can, so you can act the moment it is needed.

Taking back your decision to give your child independence is not fun, particularly for older kids. But your primary concern must be his long-term health.

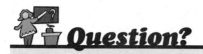 *Question?*

What if the school won't allow my child to leave the care of the nurse?
If you truly believe your child is capable and the school says no, meet with school officials and make a sales pitch. They may not be aware of new technology and how much you and your child have thought out her care plan.

You may also want to keep your school nurse in the loop. You'll still need to store supplies there, and your child will need to stop in from time to time for shots for highs or site changes or if she needs help. Tell your nurse that you'll send an e-mail once each term updating her on how your child is doing. Let her know she can call you any time. You won't want your nurse to be clueless when your child needs her.

Checking Meters, Asking Questions

Be forewarned: Your child will think that independence means her diabetes is none of your business. Now, even more than ever, it needs to be something you check on and oversee (even from a distance) each and every day.

Meter Tricks

Teens more than anyone know how to trick meters. For this reason, you'll need to keep your teen honest. At least once a day, watch as your child checks. If possible, either you or another adult should watch every check. And every day, look at the numbers in the meter and the times that are there. If your child claims the time is broken, fix it or get another meter. If your child claims he did a check on another meter, demand to see it right then.

If your child says this makes him feel as if you don't trust him, let him know that you're just looking out for his safety. If he's telling the truth, give him a day off from time to time. Let him know he can earn more independence with proven trust.

When It Doesn't Add Up

If you find that your child's actions don't match how she claims her life is going, don't be afraid to question her and don't take pat answers. As much as you want to trust your child, demand proof. If you do this from the start, it will not be confrontational. Treat it like another chore, just like taking out the trash or folding the laundry; sit down and go over the numbers with your child each day.

You'll also need to pay close attention if you see other health changes, especially rapid weight gain or loss, to make sure your child is doing well with more independence. Remember, the time will come when you set her free. It's just not completely the right time yet.

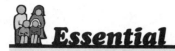

Essential

Most meters now have software for downloading numbers onto the computer. This can be a rather interesting, yet passive way for you and your child to check on how she is doing. If you don't have this software, call your meter company to get it.

Setting Your Child Free

Usually it's not until college, but there will come a time when most, if not all, of this medical responsibility becomes your child's job. That transition of power is often harder on the parent than the child, but it is a necessary transition in order for your child to live a healthy adult life.

Passing Along the Medical Team

When your child goes off to college, it may be time for him to begin seeing his medical team without you. If your child goes far away, this will be a must. But even if he is close to home and stays with his medical team, this is the time for him to visit alone. Probably, your medical team will begin meeting alone with your child for a part of each appointment during the early teen years. If they have not, ask them to begin doing that. Even though your child will be over eighteen and an adult, you can ask, with his permission, to still get a follow-up letter outlining his appointments.

The Fear of Not Knowing

Most parents of even adults with Type 1 say they are never quite able to let go of the worry and concern for their child. Talk to your adult child about how you can help her and how you'd like to stay up-to-speed with her life and her needs. Now it's her turn though; you can no longer make the plans. In the end, you will have to trust that all the years of work and dedication to your child will pay off for her as a responsible adult who cares for her diabetes well.

CHAPTER 16
Hitting the Wall: Kids and Burnout

For a child, life with diabetes can, in time, seem a dirge. Over the years, the constant schedule of blood glucose checks, insulin doses, carb counting, and, of course, a parent's nagging (i.e., "Are you low?" "Are you high?" "Did you check?") can weigh heavily on a child. Burnout is a real risk in life with diabetes, and when kids hit the wall, families can struggle in ways they never imagined. Can burnout be avoided? Probably, but not completely. Knowing how to see burnout, react to it, and work to make things better can help in the long run.

Signs and Symptoms

Let's just say this first: Parents never expect their child to burn out. They've seen the kids who have—teens who balk at daily care or younger children who flat-out give up on taking active control of their diabetes. Deep down, most parents let their egos say, "That will never be me." Well, it's time to check the ego because while some children fly through a life with diabetes without worry or care (and here's hoping yours is one of those), most children struggle at some point. You have to be understanding about this struggle: Think of how hard it is for you to keep on a diet, or to maintain a regular exercise routine. Almost all people vary from the norm (or even take a few days off) from time to time. But children with diabetes don't have

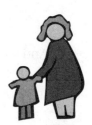

that luxury. There is no break from diabetes, not even for a day, and over the years, that's bound to take its toll.

The First Hints of Burnout

Your child has been cruising along for a few years or more, checking when needed, bolusing on time, discussing food options, and even talking openly about her diabetes for her friends and her world to hear. You live by the clock, from blood check to insulin dose to food to blood check again. You settle into thinking, "Yes, we've got this beat." And then, something starts to change.

Often, the first signs are hard for a caregiver to spot. Children are afraid, for the most part, to let their parents down. Think about it: Most parents have raved about and applauded a low A1c or a good food and bolus choice, and your children know how much you have put into helping them with this disease. Sometimes admitting she cannot "hold up her end" can be too much for a child to face.

So, kids will start to practice avoidance. They go to play across the block and "forget" the meter. You understand; you've forgotten it, too. They eat a granola bar and "forget" to bolus. You know what it's like snacking; it's easy to just gobble something down and forget you ever did.

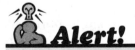

Alert!

A surprising elevation in an A1c reading can be a sign of burnout. Because kids will avoid talking about their burnout, this higher number is often the first true message a parent gets that his child is struggling.

And so, children tend to slip into burnout right under their caring and loving parents' noses. What's a parent to do? Check your ego at the door and be vigilant in looking for signs. Most parents have their egos attached to caring for their child, and with good reason. This life with diabetes takes brains and brawn, and all parents like to think they can rise to the challenge (maybe even a little better than everyone else). You see other kids who have fallen off course and cluck your tongue in disapproval. You assume your child is cruising along for one main reason: *You are a parent-hero.* As silly as that sounds, parents of children with diabetes truly are heroes. The trick is being a hero in the right way: by having an honest, open assessment of what is going on in your child's life.

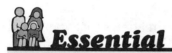

Essential

Keeping a logbook is more important than ever at this time of struggle. By forcing yourself and your child to keep one together, you'll force both of you to look honestly at the day each day. Sick of it as you may be, it works.

So, you begin to see the cracks. Missed boluses (all with excellent excuses; kids are masters at this). Forgotten blood checks. If your child used to speak openly about his disease, he may begin to keep it private.

The "I Can Do It Myself" Sign

Often, a good sign of early burnout is, ironically, something parents celebrate as a victory: a child's request to handle her diabetes on her own. This is a tricky thing. Most parents encourage their children (rightfully) to be responsible and take on duties. Life with diabetes is no different. You cheer when she does her own finger stick the first time; you call all the relatives when she gives her own shot or changes out her own pump site. But a child asking to be completely on her own—even in the teen years—is often a putting out a mayday that parents need to pick up on.

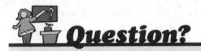 *Question?*

At what age is my child ready to do this all alone?
The long answer is he's ready once he heads to college or moves out of the house. Until then, children of all ages need their parent's support and, often, their intervention. The short answer is she'll never be ready. You'll always be your child's parent.

Another first hint is erratic blood sugar readings that your child claims not to understand or repeatedly comes up with the same "answer." If you see this, take notice. Suddenly, you notice he needed to change out sites or do shot corrections more than once a day. This is a real sign that trouble may be on the horizon, or smack in the middle of your life.

Battling Burnout

So what's a parent to do, when being a hero without an ego isn't even enough? The answer is simple (and yet like everything in diabetes, not simple at all): Take control of your child's diabetes.

A Cry for Help

While your child, even a teen, may freak out if you suddenly insist on watching her each time she checks and seeing the blood hit the meter and the meter count down, don't fret. Many children who hit burnout are crying out for help. Like anything that's hard in life, we all want to do our best, but we all need support. There's a good chance, over the years, you've pulled away from constant support of your child. This may, consciously or subconsciously, have upset her. Your child could fear a future without you helping out, a life where she pictures herself on her own. Or, he could just not want to deal with the headache of remembering to check and bolus, counting carbs, and planning out a day.

Taking Back Control

When you do decide to take back more control of the daily care, be ready to stand firm. Set some rules: "You will check your blood sugar in front of me each morning, at the nurse each day in school, and in front of me at dinner and bedtime" could be a start, if things are really dicey. "I will watch you push the buttons on your pump" might be needed as well. Don't just set these rules arbitrarily. You and your child should sit down with a professional to work them out. In most cases, your medical team will be able to help you set fair rules. If necessary, you may need to think about your child's seeing a counselor or therapist. If this is the case, make sure you work with your medical team to choose one who understands Type 1 diabetes and the issues your child faces.

Changing Things Up

Sometimes, one of the best short-term ways to fight burnout is to change things up. If your child has been on shots for a long time, this might be a good time to suggest pumping. If she's been pumping for years, it's okay to suggest going back to shots for a while. Your child may say no to those ideas, but you'll be planting a seed in her mind that she does have some control (albeit small) of the situation. You can also ask her about food choices. "Are there meals you'd like me to prepare for you? Are there changes you'd like to make in your diet?" Together with your nutritionist, you can make just about anything work. Here's another change to ponder: If one parent has been the majority stakeholder in the diabetes care, consider switching to the other caregiver.

Ask your child, if there was one thing he could change about his diabetes, what would it be? Then talk to your medical team about his answer. They may have some creative ways to help your child change or adapt at least one aspect of his care. That will show him that everyone's on his team.

Lowering Expectations

Okay, you read it. Now pick the book back up. It is important for parents to realize, as the years tick by with their child and diabetes, that children with diabetes can become perfectionists. Parents are constantly looking at what their body is doing and trying to coax it to do something else. They live by averages, A1cs, and yes, their parents' reactions to those things (see Chapter 5 for more insight into each of those). It's only a matter of time before a child takes on the need to please her parents, her medical team, and her diabetes all the time. While you never want to relax your expectations to the point of danger, you may want to remember that your child will be working at caring for this disease every hour of her life until a cure is found.

If you are a parent who has a child check more than seven or eight times a day, lowering your expectations might mean having him cut back to six, or even five. Your medical team can help you look at your child's schedule and come up with an agreed-upon daily care plan that cuts back but is still healthful and appropriate. Compromise may be your best friend here.

It's Okay Not to Like It

Your child hears it all the time: "You'll be fine once you're regulated." Or "I hear it's a very controllable disease." Or "At least it's not something life threatening." We all flinch at those remarks, but to children who struggle and yet never seem to feel as though they've completely beaten diabetes, those comments can be emotional bombshells.

It's important to validate your child's discouragement. Rather than "Oh, come on! You can do it!" consider being honest, to a point, with your child. Diabetes is a difficult, all-encompassing disease that would burn out the best of us. Encourage your child to accept that truth, and then, challenge him to change it. Point out that in life, the challenging times make us who we are. Promise him to do all you can to bring him around. Never, ever, scold him or tell him he should be used to it all by now (plenty of strangers will have said that already). Instead, allow him to take ownership of a tough situation, and then lead him to a better place with it.

When Nothing Works

You take over control and work to help your child feel as if she can make some changes. You talk to the social worker and get good tips. And yet, burnout keeps rearing its head. What's a family to do?

Punish or Protect?

Punishment is not the answer; protection is. It's tempting to set limits and dole out punishments to try to force your child into compliance. But most children already feel punished by diabetes; adding to that will only push them deeper into their state. However, setting limits with consequences is acceptable.

Let's say your son has been "forgetting" to bolus at morning snack at school every day. It's perfectly acceptable to set limits that have to do with his safety. In this case, you'd give him two choices: no more snack in the morning (if not medically needed), or an additional blood sugar check two hours after the snack so that a correction can be made before he has been high for too long without checking.

It's *not* okay to take that same situation and say, "You're off the Internet until you remember to bolus for a week." It is okay to say, "Because you have forgotten to do your lunch blood sugar check three times, you have to go to the school nurse again to do it for the next month." Agree that after that month, you'll let your child try to win his freedom again.

Counseling: Finding the Best

You've worked with your medical team and talked to your support group, but you still struggle daily with your once-compliant child. It's probably time for more help. Finding the right counselor and helping your child use that person well is a challenge, but it is one worth taking.

Not Everyone Is an Expert

By now, you know that just about everyone out there thinks he or she knows a lot about diabetes. By now, you also know that *thinks* is the relative word here. Misconceptions about diabetes, particularly Type 1, are rampant. Counselors are no exception.

If and when you decide your child needs regular counseling, be painstaking in your choice. Talk first to your medical team's social worker, not only to help you find a therapist with some background in diabetes and/or chronic illnesses in children, but also to help you find one who would be a good match for your child. Your social worker should be familiar with the counselors in your area and able to refer you to one who is taking new patients.

If your social worker does not know of a therapist close to you, ask if he will at least help you develop a list of questions to ask any counselor you interview (and the answers you should want to hear). Even better, ask if he'll call a counselor on your child's behalf to discuss the situation and your child's needs and help you decide if this is the right person to help your child.

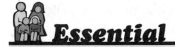 *Essential*

If a counselor seems perfect to you on paper, but your child feels differently, respect her feeling and make a change. Your child will need to feel completely comfortable with her counselor. Encourage your child to give a counselor at least three meetings before deciding.

You'll also want to make sure your counselor is open to constructive ideas from you and your medical team. In the end, while the counselor will help your child learn to cope with burnout, you are still the diabetes expert.

Close to Home

Although you may be willing to drive for hours to see a great pediatric endocrinology team, a counselor should be close to home. Your child may be seeing the counselor as much as once a week, and you'll want this to have as little impact on his life as possible. Time in a car both ways can add up.

In order for your child to buy into this help, you'll want it to be as noninvasive as possible. That also means finding a therapist who will meet with your child not just after school, but after (or before) sports or other activities your child loves.

Of course, this is no small task. If you come up empty, ask your child's school psychologist to work with you to find some good leads. But again, don't just go on what she says. Make sure you and your social worker know this counselor understands your child's unique needs.

Other Places Your Child Can Heal

Counseling alone may not be enough for your child. Even if she doesn't need counseling, there are places, events, and programs that may help your child come around to once again living in peace with her diabetes.

"They're All Just Like Me"

Whether it's a support group or a diabetes camp, as discussed in Chapter 13, your child will find some peace in spending time at a place where everyone is just like her. Diabetes camp is probably your best choice, and in some areas, camps offer year-round programs and even quick weekend programs for kids to get a dose of help.

You may also be able to find a few other kids your child's age in your general area. Finding your child a local "diabetes buddy" can be a big help. Much as parents like to think they are the ones who know their children best, there's no one to talk this through with better than another child living the same life.

Role Model

If you're dealing with a teen or even a preteen, you may want to allow him to participate in some events that make him feel like a role model. Kids love being looked up to, and little kids really look up to bigger kids with diabetes. Be careful, though: Don't put your child in a position of having another person to "let down" if he doesn't take care of his diabetes. Rather, ask your child if he would mentor a younger child. Tell him the younger child could learn a lot from him—and then see where it goes.

You can also allow her to go public with her disease. This is a personal decision, and again, care is needed with the handling of this. While some children are empowered by being heard in a public way, others find it puts too much pressure on them. Bring your child to an event where a child her age talks about her diabetes and then see how she reacts. If speaking out empowers her to move past the point of burnout, fantastic. If not, at least she will have learned something.

The Age Question

Some experts think that burnout comes only to teens, and others think it occurs in time. If your child is diagnosed at a young age, is he more likely to be hit with burnout?

Issues of the Young

Young children tend not to burn out on diabetes, and that makes sense. While the idea of a life with constant intervention seems horrible to grownups, little ones don't truly understand the concept of time. Think of how your child always thinks a holiday is "tomorrow," or asks if a week will be over in a minute. That concept of time helps her deal with the day-to-day reality of diabetes.

Little ones are pleasers; they want Mom and Dad to be happy with them. This leads many tiny kids with diabetes to take on things like finger pokes, shots, or infusion site setup help at a young age. You are their idol and their greatest love. They'll do anything to please you.

But the very young grow up, and often, years of battling diabetes in a brave and unquestionable way come to a screeching halt. For all the kids diagnosed at twelve who feel a bit overwhelmed by thirteen, by this point children diagnosed at a very young age can have as much as a decade (or more) of diabetes experience under their belt.

By the time they are teenagers, little ones often have no memory of life without diabetes. This can be stressful, leaving the child yearning for what that feeling is like. It's a hard thing for a parent to answer: What's it like *not* to have diabetes? It can be heartbreaking to hear, since parents often try not to remember that their child has no recall of life without diabetes. Make sure you let your child know that while he may not know that feeling now, it is your deepest hope that someday, in his future, he'll feel just that.

Older Kids

That's not to say it's easier being diagnosed at an older age. Preteens and teens are at a rough patch of life anyway. The last thing they want is to be perceived as different; the last thing they are interested in is being tethered even tighter to their parents. Yet here they are, struggling with a disease most kids have never heard of and living a life that demands constant parent intervention. Burnout can come hard and fast.

With a newly diagnosed preteen or teen, it is vitally important that you find her help and support right away. Try, as best you can, to show her that while this may change some things in her life, most will remain the same. She'll still play sports. She'll still go to school. She'll still date and get her driver's license. If she can adapt to this and be open with you about how she feels, you can help her find a way to feel at least some freedom while under your constant care.

Young or older, if your child knows that burnout happens to the best kids, he should be able to talk to you early, and in the end, perhaps you'll be able to offset some of the hard times.

CHAPTER 17

Hitting the Wall: Parent/Caregiver Burnout

Y ou are your child's rock. Through this challenging time, you've stood strong; learning all you can and adjusting your life to make your child's life less impacted by diabetes. You don't mind; it's your job as a parent. But in time, many parents yearn for a time when they didn't know the carb content of every food on earth, when they could go to bed at night not thinking about blood sugar levels. Yes, burnout hits parents, too.

Signs and Symptoms

It's hard for a parent or caregiver to admit to burnout. Your child is your life, and you would literally give an arm or a leg to rid her of this disease or at least make her life easier while she struggles with it. Admitting that you're sick of it—or that you're slacking off in your drive to keep up with it—is hard to do, but sometimes you must. The never-ending, moment-to-moment intervention that diabetes demands of you as a parent can pare you down to a nub. No good parent wants to let his child down, and burning out, when you don't even have the disease, can feel like the ultimate cop-out.
Knowing the symptoms and realizing you are not alone can help.

Cracks in the Foundation
All parents start out vigilant. Your supply drawers are meticulous; your logbooks could be framed as

examples to all others. You're ahead on your prescription refill needs, and you never, ever forget to carry along a fast-acting glucose no matter where you go. But time ticks on and, eventually, diabetes becomes a routine. The problem is, unlike other routines, it is not a welcome one. So, over the years, you just get sick of it.

Think of it this way: The phases of a child's life can be challenging, but they change. While the routine of feeding, changing, and helping a baby get to sleep can be monotonous over time, you know one day that baby will be a toddler and you'll be on to other routines. Diabetes is just not that way. For as long as your child is in your care, these needs will be here.

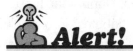

Alert!

Super parents may be more susceptible to burnout. If you're writing and rewriting the notes in your child's logbook, talk to your endocrinologist about ways you can back off and still give excellent care. Don't set your own bar too high.

We start to see the cracks. It becomes easier not to write in the logbook every day. You begin to eyeball a plate of food and guesstimate a carb count. You open the butter compartment in the refrigerator only to realize you've run out of insulin. Little things begin to fall apart. You are burning out. Most parents don't want to accept that but facing it head-on and finding ways to re-ignite your dedication (and not head back to burnout again) will only help your child.

Feelings of Guilt

As burnout creeps in, a parent usually first feels guilty. Your child is the one who has to live with diabetes 24/7. Your child has to bear so much more than you, how could you ever get sick of helping him? The answer to these feelings of guilt is simple: You're only human.

The best thing to do about your guilt is face it and move past it. When you had a child, you signed on to a lifetime of love, care, and support. But never did you visualize constant blood checks, injections, pump site changes, and carb-effect studies. Parenting a child with diabetes is far from easy. Everyone is going to burn out from time to time. It's what you do when that burnout hits that really matters.

Avoiding Burnout

Take this little pill and you'll never burn out on your diabetes care routine. If only it were that easy. Avoiding burnout can be tough because most parents don't realize it's an issue until they've hit it head-on. So the first step to avoiding burnout is accepting that there's a real chance you might face it one day. Put down that ego again and realize you are not invincible; you have your own needs and desires and feelings, as much as you may feel you should not for the sake of your child.

A Team Effort

The next step is simple to say and yet so hard to put into practice. Make sure you and your spouse are equal partners in the care of your child. If you are a single parent, sign on another caring adult to be your partner.

The spouse issue can be tricky. As we discussed in Chapter 9, each parent can take on a unique role, almost like the 1950s-style parents Ward and June Cleaver, once a child is diagnosed. If you are reading this book, there's a good chance you're the June of the situation: taking total control of the diabetes and all of its needs so everyone else can be comfortable and cared for. The problem is that as you (subliminally) refuse to trust anyone else with the care of your child, you cut off your own lifeline. You need to have people who can take over and give you a break.

If you are early in the stages of learning to care for your child, make sure to include this person—a spouse, a relative, or a friend—in as many appointments and training sessions as possible. While it's easy for one spouse to attend these meetings and hand the information to the other, the couple that attends appointments together naturally takes a more cooperative role in caring for the child.

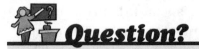 ***Question?***

What if I have no one to help?
For single parents without much family, this can be a challenge. Reach out to a trusted friend and ask him to be your partner. You'd say yes if he asked you, wouldn't you? Don't be afraid to ask for help.

No matter how much you cringe at his or her style, allow your spouse or partner to take over total care half the time. Sure, you do shots differently than he does, but it doesn't matter. Sharing the daily tasks will help you not be alone in this job.

What about the full-time working spouse? She can still do a bedtime check, nighttime check, and even count the carbs at dinner (or breakfast when she is home). It is too easy to just make it your job. Make the extra effort to make it someone else's too.

Take a Vacation

Many parents or caregivers struggle with this issue. If my child never has a vacation, they reason, why should I? There are two simple reasons: because you need to, and because you can. You are now basically working as a full-time, always on-call nurse to your child. A vacation from that, even if it's just a weekend off with friends or one day and night in the city, will refresh you and remind you of what it's like to live life without thinking about diabetes all the time.

For the lucky families that have loving grandparents or aunts and uncles involved, this could be a vacation for both caretakers. But if you are like a majority of parents, you don't have anyone beyond your own home to help care for a child overnight. Don't let that stop you: Take a weekend alone and then let your spouse take one. Just getting away, at least once a year, is key.

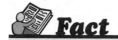 **Fact**

Many diabetes camps offer winter weekends for kids. These camps provide a chance for parents to get away while knowing their child is in good hands. One such center is the Barton Center in Massachusetts: Visit their web site at *www.bartoncenter.org.*

It's an unspoken rule that sending kids to diabetes camp in the summer is as much for the parents as it is for the kids. A week or two at camp gives the caretaker time to relax, regroup, and face another year of caring for her child. Do try to convince your child (and yourself) that diabetes camp is the way to go.

Mini-breaks

If a vacation is out of the question, find a regular mini-break for yourself. Join a book group. Take up tennis. Try golf. Book a spa treatment every other week. Take a long walk each evening. Whatever it is you choose, agree with your spouse or fellow caretaker that during that activity, you will not be contacted about diabetes, unless it is a true crisis. A weekly mini-break can refresh you and also give you something to anticipate. It can also remind you that there's a world out there, and you are still part of it.

When you do take your time, put the cell phone on vibrate. Ask your spouse or fellow caretaker to hold off on calling you. Not only will this give you a much needed break, it will force him to take control and force you to allow him to do so.

Battling Burnout

When it hits, burnout can be devastating. The guilt, the anger, the loneliness can strike a parent or caregiver hard. Sometimes, a quick fix brings you around. Other times, more help is needed. Taking the right steps at the right time will help you come around.

Accepting Where You Are

Most times, the burned-out parent has allowed diabetes (justifiably so) to take over her life. She may have given up something she loves; some parents of very young children even put a career on hold. Many have let their marriage fall into a state of disrepair. The combination of stress, worry, anger, and task-sharing issues can push a couple pretty far. The best first step toward moving out of that hole is to accept that you are in it.

Sounds easy, but it's not. Parents just don't want to fail, and like any humans, they don't want to look closely and realize that their own actions may have helped get them to this point. The parent who can say out loud "I've let this go too far," or "I've set myself up for failure here," is the parent who will come out of burnout ready to begin anew.

Don't Play the Blame Game

Adults can be great at assigning blame. The reason you have to take on all the diabetes care, you claim, is that your spouse just does not care. The reason you've never taken on any responsibility is that your spouse just does not trust you. The reason you're down in the dumps is that your mother-in-law won't have your daughter for sleepovers anymore.

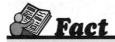 **Fact**

Diabetes can sometimes hurt others around you, too. If you have a good friend or relative who has cut back on a relationship with your child because of fear, chances are she is hurting too. Offer to help her change that.

Learn now: Blame does no good. The situation is a complicated one, and even if you do have a point in some cases, pointing fingers does not move you forward. Rather, look at the situation and figure out how you can change it. Ask your mother-in-law what keeps her from hosting sleepovers anymore? You may be surprised by the answer. If it's her thinking that you don't trust her, you can help her change that with training and education.

With a spouse or partner, it can be trickier. The diagnosis of a chronic disease can throw a wrench into even the best relationship, and one person in the couple experiencing burnout can only hurt it more. People tend to lash out at those who are closest and to get bitter about things the other spouse may not even realize. A sit-down with your spouse to admit that you're in over your head and need support is a brave step. You may be surprised at what you hear. While some spouses who are not providing hands-on care may be practicing avoidance, others report that they feel pushed away by the dominant care-taking parent. If your spouse is the latter, you'll need to take a deep breath and realize you have work to do to let that spouse into the diabetes care equation. If your spouse is the avoidance type, you've got a whole different issue. Either way, make sure you go about this discussion away from the ears of your child (he feels enough stress and guilt without hearing his disease may have pitted parent against parent) and in a way that is not confrontational.

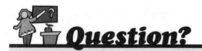 **Question?**

What if I cannot be calm about this?
Then it's time to bring a professional in. You would not be the first couple to seek expert help in working out this situation, and you won't be the last. Find a counselor and begin addressing the issue.

By putting blame aside and just addressing the situation and your desire to change it, you'll find that both sides can be heard, responded to, and, you hope, made happy again with tweaks and changes in the daily care routine and relationship.

Make It a Real Plan

It's not enough here to say, "Okay, I'll help out more." You and your fellow caregiver need to sit down and hash out a real plan with real expectations. You need to contract your plan, just as you do with your child and her diabetes care. For instance, if you feel your spouse needs to be more on board, you might write out, "Both parents will attend next four endocrinology appointments." Or "Spouses will alternate weekends of being in charge of shots, insulin, and carb counting." Write down, too, what you *won't* do. "Neither caregiver will criticize the methods of the other" is a good start. You don't have to frame it or cross-stitch it, but putting it in writing, as always, makes you think it through and makes it real.

When Nothing Works

You sit down and talk it out. You write out a plan and try to stick to it. You reach out to friends and support groups for feedback. And yet, you still feel as if you're drowning in the daily tasks of diabetes. It's time to take more drastic action.

Baby Steps

First off, are you trying to change too quickly? Working your way out of burnout may be about baby steps. You simply cannot change years of habit and patterning in a day or even a fortnight. Consider making a list of what you'd like to change and then working through the issues one at a time. Baby steps will get you there, and even if it takes more time than you'd like, at least you'll be moving toward your goal. For instance, if your dream is to get back to a point where you are focusing on diabetes with all the attention it needs, a good first step might be "I will keep a logbook again." Commit to that one act and give it a week or two. Once you are back in the swing of keeping the logbook, add the next goal: "I will do a fasting blood glucose check this month," and see if you can do it. One by one, take on the re-entry needed to get back up to speed.

Find Something New

The same strategy applies for helping others adapt to what you want. If you reach out to your sister and tell her you need her to learn about diabetes, don't expect her to read the entire guide and pass your approval with soaring colors the first week. Rather, go slowly. Ask her to come to a support meeting. Encourage her to read up on Internet sites and reach out to other aunts of children with diabetes. Give it time. Perhaps just seeing that someone is willing to try for you and your child will help bring you around.

New and Improved Support

If it's been a while since you've been to your support group, it's time to check back in. If you've never felt you've needed support before, now's the time to begin. Hearing that others feel the same way you do can be like an elixir. Check in with local organizations to find support. If you are far away from any in-person support, check it out online. (See Chapter 12 for ideas and details on support for parents.)

You should also talk to your social worker. The medical team is there for you as much as for your child, and they've seen it all before. They can be a great resource not only for ways to battle burnout, but to help you assess how deep you are, and what kind of help you might need to move past it.

Counseling: When and Where?

At a certain point, you may want to consider counseling for yourself, your spouse, and perhaps eventually your entire family. Your child's diagnosis can trigger depression, and your burnout could be a symptom. If you've tried everything and still cannot rally, it's time to move to professional help.

When You Know You Need It

Obviously, clear signs of depression such as thoughts of suicide, rapid weight gain or loss, or an inability to socialize as you once did need to be addressed immediately. But the signs that you need to see a counselor can be more subtle.

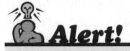 **Alert!**

While it would be nice to find a counselor who has dealt with parents of children with chronic diseases, you don't need to be as picky as you were in finding the one for your child. A good therapist whom you bond with will suffice.

If you simply can no longer face the day-to-day routine of caring for your child, no matter how hard you try to start again, you need to seek professional help. Your child needs you—for a good long time—as their guide, helper, and adviser.

Without the constant support of a caring and healthy parent, a child has less chance of long-term success fighting diabetes. Again, don't feel like a failure. Your willingness to take the time to seek counseling to heal yourself is a great effort for your child. If you find you've lost interest in all the other things you used to do, counseling is needed as well.

Where to Go

As you did when you were looking for a counselor for your child, check first with your medical team and social worker to ask them if they have any recommendations in your area. Find one as close to home or work as possible. You'll need to see this counselor for some time, so making it convenient only makes sense. Besides, you've been stressed out enough in life at this point; having to travel a great distance might only make things worse. Try to find a way to make it work without having to worry about your child while you have your appointments. If you can find a friend nearby who can watch your child, or if your spouse can help out by being home for the appointments, it will free you up to focus on yourself, which will free you up to focus again on your child and their health.

How to Escape

Sometimes, you'll need to just escape from the day-to-day tedious-ness of diabetes care. There is nothing wrong or abnormal about that desire, you are a parent or caregiver, but you are human as well. You will occasionally feel the need to get away. By planning ahead and using good sense, you may be able to do just that.

Far and Away

There's a legend of a couple with a small child with diabetes who cruised to Tahiti for a week (if you're reading this, you know who you are). Their diabetes-world friends marveled at their ability to make it work. It was no small feat. They found a college-age nursing student who had had Type 1 since she was a small girl. They hired her as a sitter once a week for a year, which helped their child and the sitter bond. They then purchased two wireless communication devices, such as a BlackBerry, and a computer program and trained the sitter so they'd be able to check in regularly on how their child was doing. Then, one spring day, they cruised.

Sure, it wasn't easy, and it took a major investment of smarts, time, and money. But do you think as they clicked margarita glasses at sunset, they whined?

A long trip *can* happen, if you have the chutzpah. Diabetes camp is a great way to make it work easily; finding a trained sitter you know well is tougher but still possible (admittedly with a bit of luck).

Short Trips

There's also the concept of just getting away for a bit. What about an overnight in a lovely hotel right in your own town? If you have a friend or family member you trust, pack your bag and spend twenty-four hours close enough not to worry but far enough to get away from it. Book a spa treatment; bring a book (but not one on diabetes!).

Allow yourself one full day and night of leisure. See if you don't come back refreshed—and, having trusted your friend or family member that one night, you may be on your way to that long trip. Remember, it starts with baby steps.

CHAPTER 18

Teen Issues

D
iabetes takes on a whole new life in the teen years. Whether you are dealing with a new diagnosis or continuing a long-running battle with the disease, everything that makes teens the unique creatures they are—hormones, social pressures, lifestyle changes, a smattering of arrogance—complicates the diabetes structure. It takes patience, adaptation, and sometimes a whole lot of help and support to get through those years. (Okay and maybe a little prayer.)

Attitude Changes

If your child has had diabetes for a number of years, you may have been lulled into a sense that she is one of the few who will never struggle with the disease. If your child is new to diabetes, you may hope that his lifetime of cooperation and good deeds means this will be a snap, too. But often, attitudes change and so does self-care in diabetes.

Long-Timers

For kids who have been dealing with diabetes for a long time—say, more than four years—the teen years can be particularly difficult. You start with the public perception ("Oh, she's had it for so long; it must be second nature by now") and add the fact that teens just

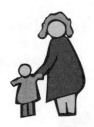

don't like to conform to much of anything an adult suggests, and you've got a tricky diabetes situation.

Part of the issue can be, as discussed in the last chapter, burnout, but it can also be your teen wanting to conform to her peers. Let's face it, all kids grow past that phase of always wanting to please you (and other important adults in their lives) to thinking they know just a wee bit more (okay, a whole lot more) than anyone else. When that mind-set comes into play with curfews or homework habits, it can be stressful enough. But when it has to do with managing a life-threatening disease, it's a whole new level of worry for parents or caregivers.

Noticing a Change

You start to see the shift, usually, toward the late part of the middle school years, just about the time teens are truly becoming teens. The girl who once simply clipped her pump to her belt buckle and let it hang out there now painstakingly finds ways to hide it. The boy who whipped out his meter on the sidelines at Little League now wants to check only in the car and not bring his meter with him. Kids who once simply complied with your every order (do a bolus; check your blood; treat a low) begin to question or, even worse, avoid you.

The worrisome part about teens who have had diabetes for a number of years is that they've learned the tricks of the trade. It takes a few years to start contemplating how to trick your parents and even your equipment when it comes to diabetes. Most newly diagnosed teens don't consider manipulating a meter to show a different number or not to check at all, yet long-timers have been known to do this.

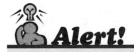

Alert!

A first sign of manipulation is when a child suddenly does all bolusing and checking out of your sight. This secrecy is often a sign that your child is experiencing burnout. Keep a watchful eye on the process, particularly in the teen years.

Long-timers, too, may suffer from the rest of the world being "over" their disease. If in their first years friends donated to their "walk to cure" team or offered to help, that support may have waned because, even though there will never be a "remission" or a let-down in their fight, the rest of the world tends to move on. If this is the case, try to find a new way to make your child feel as though people care. (See Chapter 20 for more ideas.) This feeling that the rest of the world has moved on could lead your teen to feeling as if he should move on, too, when in fact, diabetes never gets easier. Rather, it just changes.

Newbie Teens

Kids with diabetes debate all the time whether it is easier to be a teen who simply does not recall what it's like to live without diabetes, or to be older when you begin this new life? It's almost like the quandary of the chicken and the egg. Some teens think that if you don't know any different way of life, it has to be easier to accept, while others say that not knowing any different way makes it harder to accept. Whichever side of the discussion you come down on, everyone agrees that adapting to a new disease and new lifestyle smack in the middle of the teen years can be rough.

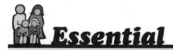 *Essential*

If your child is diagnosed as a teen, make sure you learn to give shots and blood checks as well, even if your teen never wants you to do it. Even if you never give one, you need to understand the process to help make it better for your child.

First off, your teen is not in your constant care. While a small child with diabetes tends to be in the capable hands of a caring adult at all times, teens are more on their own. They're at sports practice, hanging out with friends, or just in their room with the door shut. They're beginning to create their own world, and the invasion of the D-Parent chanting, "Are you low? Are you low?" can be a shock.

Younger children are more willing to share their story with the world, too. You really cannot come into your child's middle or high school to do a cute show-and-tell on diabetes using a teddy bear and a children's book. (Well, you could, but your child would never speak to you again, and other parents would think you were nuts.) Your teen won't want to scream it from the mountains (or possibly even whisper it at the lunch table), and yet, people need to know. So, spreading the word of your teen's new diagnosis can be challenging.

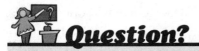

Question?

Can my teen keep diabetes a secret?
This is a dangerous situation and needs to be addressed. The people around your teen—her friends, teachers, coaches—need to know she has diabetes. If it is common knowledge, it is not a big deal. Insist on public knowledge.

Work with your medical team to find a compromise for your teen. Explain to her that once people know, it will be old news. Ask your team to explain that for her safety, people simply need to know.

The "Cool" Factor

Can having diabetes be cool? That's a stretch. But ironically, while most teens want to deny it, they can also find that accepting it and being a role model could be cool. This is not easy to make happen, but if you can do it, you're a long way into surviving the teen years.

When It's Not Cool

Teens, for the most part, feel anything out of the norm is not cool. So at school or at the park, they may dislike having to check their blood sugars, wear a pump, or take a shot; they may even be embarrassed. Talk to your teen about ways to do what he has to do discreetly; approach this discussion with care. Diabetes is a part of him, and you don't want him to think that he has to keep that part compartmentalized.

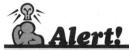

Alert!

Never force a child to do blood checks or shots in a restroom or away from people. Telling her to "hide" her diabetes sends a subliminal, dangerous, and false message that she should be ashamed of herself or that diabetes is something she should be ashamed of.

Teens may think that going low isn't very cool either, so many purposely run their blood sugars higher. It's hard for your teen to completely avoid lows when he's in tight control, but try to encourage him to know how to treat them quickly and easily. Keeping candy in his pocket is a simple solution. Be sure to remind him that highs are not cool either; he can be more irritable, unreasonable, and even mess up in school while running high. Help him remember how much better he feels when his blood sugars are in a tighter range. In the end, try to help him realize that a few lows are worth avoiding the constant irritation of running high.

Making It Cool

While it's not easy, it is possible to find ways to make living with diabetes a bit cooler. With creativity and cooperation, you can find some ways.

The biggest obstacle some parents face with teens is wearing a medical alert bracelet. When your kids are little, they'll clip it on and never complain. As they get older, they may ask for a neater one: for girls, a glittery one; for boys, usually a sporty one. But once they hit the teen years, they just don't want to wear one at all.

Ironically, this is one of the most vital times to wear one. Explain to your teen that while she may think that no one needs to check to see if she has diabetes, this is the time it could most be needed. She'll be driving with friends, off at events and parties, and not everyone will always know her story. Although she may think she can depend on her friends, the truth is, she can never depend on another person to deliver the message of her special needs in an emergency.

 Essential

Most medical teams agree that wearing a medic alert during the teen years is non-negotiable. Having the team, rather than you, the parents, explain that to your child may help your case. Ask your endocrinologist to point out why the medical alert is a necessity, giving you needed backup.

So, the cool factor here may come with a price tag. Ask your child what he would consider wearing as a medic alert. Then, buy it, regardless of whether it is from Tiffany's or is any other high-priced item. In the end, your peace of mind will be worth the cost. One warning: Never give medical alert jewelry as a holiday or birthday gift. Nothing about diabetes should be a "gift," and deep down, no child really wants that identification, no matter how expensive or beautiful it is.

Teens may feel it is rather dorky to have to carry a meter around as well. Again, make the investment into something—anything— she'd be willing to use to carry her meter.

Cool Outreach

Cool can also come in the form of making a difference, too. Teens are at a point in their life where they not only need to gather community service hours but a good show of fundraising or advocacy can separate them from the crowd when it comes to filling out their college applications. Talk to your child about the opportunities kids with diabetes have to make a difference (see Chapter 20 for details).

Another way to make it cool is to find a place where your child is the same as everyone else. As discussed in Chapter 13, diabetes camps are ideal for this. Nothing brings a kid around more than being one of many rather than being alone.

Driving

Okay, now that you've caught your breath, it's time to think about teens and driving. Because as stressful as it is for any parent to train his child to drive and then send him on his way, parents of kids with diabetes win the prize.

The Law and Diabetes

Yes, you can get a driver's license if you have diabetes. But in some states, you may be required to submit some sort of medical documentation beforehand. In Texas, for example, all new drivers are asked if they have diabetes and if they've had severe lows or complications. If you answer yes to any of these questions, you may be required to submit documentation from your doctor.

It is important to let your teen know from the start that while getting a low is not their fault, driving while low can be punishable by law. If a person with diabetes has a car accident while low (or extremely high), he or she can be held accountable. Explain to your child that driving while low is much like driving while drunk. Her instincts and reactions will be impaired, and because it is her responsibility to check before driving (or during driving on a long trip), the law may hold her accountable.

How to Start

Setting rules before your teen ever gets behind the wheel is the right way to start. It's safe to say that every person with diabetes (particularly those who experience lows or have trouble detecting lows) need to check his or her blood sugar before even starting the engine. Set a higher driving target range than your usual range. In other words, if you consider 70–130 within range, make 100–180 your driving range.

Set time limits on how often your child needs to check her blood sugar levels when driving. For instance, if she is heading out on a long trip, or just planning on cruising around town with her friends, you may want to have her check her blood sugar every two hours.

Your teen driver with diabetes should always have a fast-acting carb in the car. A juice box or two or glucose tabs will suffice. Encourage him to pull over when he feels low (and make sure to teach him, from the get-go, how and where to pull over safely on any road).

When to Say No

Driving a car is a privilege, one that your child has more responsibility to earn than most kids. Like irresponsible kids who speed or drink and drive, teens with diabetes who do not follow their special rules agreed on by their family and medical team must not be allowed to drive.

So what actions warrant taking away the car keys? If your teen is not following the rules and checking and treating her blood sugars before driving and during long drives, you've got to ground her because, like it or not, this action is for the safety of the general public as well as your child.

Beyond that, you may want to set some other rules that are deal breakers, such as manipulating meters or otherwise lying about blood sugars (or not checking. It's all about trust. Trusting your child behind the wheel of a car is a big deal, and if she betrays your trust in general, it will take time (non-driving time that is) for her to win it back.

You'll want to practice what you preach, too. You are not alone: All parents are fearful when their children begin to drive, with or without diabetes. Your child may be motivated enough about the chance to drive that he'll surprise you and be responsible and careful.

Alcohol

The issues that endanger all teens are doubly dangerous to teens with diabetes. For this reason, parents often begin educating their children about these issues at a younger age than most. It's never too early to begin laying the groundwork for your teen to understand their risks and the ramifications of dangerous behavior as compared to children without diabetes.

The Physiology of Drinking

It's a fact: Drinking alcohol lowers your blood sugar. No matter how "in control" your child's diabetes may be, it might only take one night of drinking to send her on an ambulance ride, or worse. Talking to your child frankly and honestly about drinking is a must, as uncomfortable as it may be for both of you.

Although you'd really like to just say "don't drink!" that's not dealing with reality. The better option is to tell your child that you do not allow or condone underage drinking, but that you'd rather he understands the way to do it than to do it wrong if he is going to sneak in a drinking night.

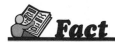 **Fact**

Alcohol is not a never-in-your-life thing for diabetes. The American Diabetes Association says that used in moderation (no more than two drinks a day for an adult) and with food, alcohol is fine for adults with diabetes. Tell your child the time will come.

You'll want to share this information with your child, while stressing that their best option is no alcohol at all.

Pushing Abstinence

So how do you walk the line of urging a child not to drink but sharing with them best practices if they do drink? As always, involve the experts. Have your endocrinologist or Certified Diabetes Educator talk with her about alcohol and back it up with a talk (or ten or twenty) of your own. Drive home the fact that drinking alcohol with diabetes is tricky; it takes planning, counting, and attention. Ironically, alcohol can rob a person (particularly a teen) of the ability to do all three of those things. Tell your child that eating carbs along with drinking is a good idea, as is testing blood sugars every hour.

Alcohol's Long-Term Effects

Be honest about the long-term effects of alcohol on people with diabetes. If diabetes is not well-controlled, long-term drinking can increase the chances of complications such as eye damage. A hangover, complete with vomiting, can throw off insulin absorption enough to require a trip to the emergency room. That's not a fun short-term effect.

You may also want to consider allowing your child to call his endocrinologist if he gets into a bad situation with alcohol. If the endocrinologist on call can help him get out of a potentially dangerous situation, it's better than the alternative. But do stress to your teen: If he calls you because of a bad alcohol situation, you will not yell at him or ground him. There will be consequences of some kind, but the alternative is much worse. Create a plan where he can reach out for help before it's too late.

Sex and Other Traps

It's hard enough talking about sex with your teen. Adding diabetes to it makes it even more complicated but even more important. Your child will need to understand all about sex well before she considers it, and you hope that she will be open to discussing it with you as she grows.

Boys and Sex

Once upon a time, it was said that all boys with diabetes would grow up to have erectile dysfunction. Today's blatant ads for medications to treat that condition do little to erase that perception. But the truth today is that with the better insulin, meters, and, therefore, control that kids experience, erectile dysfunction is not necessarily in your son's future.

Your son will need to hear that, because, thanks to those same commercials, he may hear talk about it or even be teased about it in school. When you talk sex with your son with diabetes, be sure to explain to him what causes this in men with diabetes, and why he can be different from those men.

Then, you need to talk about what having sex means to a boy with diabetes. This may take some backup, and this is yet another reason to have an endocrinologist he likes and trusts. Because—surprise, surprise—sex burns carbs and that could mean lows.

Girls and Sex

Girls, too, burn carbs during sex and need to learn how to prepare with a blood check and a snack (doesn't that sound spontaneous?). So, they need to be doubly careful.

A pregnancy with diabetes must be planned out and treated with care. Your daughter needs to realize that most women with diabetes who have babies begin taking extra care and running even tighter blood sugars before they get pregnant.

Getting pregnant without planning ahead may not only mean trouble for your daughter, if blood sugars are extremely erratic, it could mean trouble for the baby, in the way of birth defects. No parents want their teen to have sex. Encourage her to use diabetes as even more of a reason *not* to give into pressure to have sex.

But you need to let your daughter know that, should she decide she is going to have sex, you'd rather her be open and let you (or her medical team) help her use birth control. The alternative, an unwanted pregnancy, is so much worse.

Drugs

There's an old wives' tale that endocrinologists like to tell teens with diabetes that marijuana is a better alternative to drinking. While it may be true that pot does not lower the blood sugar as quickly as alcohol, it is in no way true that it is a viable option. First, there's the whole illegal thing. Beyond that, pot impairs the decision-making process and causes "munchies." Lows and highs are just as much a danger with pot as they are with alcohol. In fact, all drug use should be avoided. Talk to your teen, again, about why this is more important to her than to anyone without diabetes. Perhaps the added risk will scare them. Again, drive home a plan that means if your child makes a bad choice, she can call you or her medical team for help.

Recognizing a Cry for Help

It can be easy in the teen years not to pick up on the first hints of trouble with your child. There's so much going on anyway: new independence, fewer restrictions, tougher classes, and even new friends. But parents and caregivers need to keep a close watch on their teens to help steer them away from trouble in "diabetes land."

Fantasy Versus Reality

Your child, and you, may end up with two distinctly different frames of reference: fantasy and reality. In fantasy, your child is completely compliant with their diabetes care. He doesn't mind blood checks; he is careful when he is out with friends. Your child tells you he's fine on his own and that he is now ready to take on diabetes by himself. The teen years are absolutely not the time for this. (See Chapter 15 for a detailed discussion on independence and timing.)

This is tough because as a parent, your instinct tells you to encourage your teen to work on his own; he is growing up and spreading his wings. But most pediatric endocrinologists agree that teens need direct parental involvement in diabetes care up until the time they go to college and sometimes longer than that.

For your child, the fantasy may be that he doesn't really have diabetes; or it really does not require the care that you insist it does.

In some cases, sadly, this can all come to a head in the emergency room. More than one parent has found out for the first time that their teen has been noncompliant after they develop diabetic ketoacidosis, a life-threatening condition described in Chapter 5. Others are lucky enough to find out by an elevated A1c. If you do discover this way, keep in mind: In your teen's fantasy world, this may be the first time he actually realizes he's been off the program.

Weight Loss and a Bad Self-Image

Teens, too, can suffer from eating disorders and depression. If you notice your teen is running high blood sugars, you may want to explore the possibility of an eating disorder.

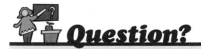 *Question?*

My child eats a lot. How can she have a disorder?
Diabulimia is the act of eating and then not bolusing for it, which allows the person to eat all he or she wants and still lose weight because of the lack of insulin. This is a dangerous situation.

As for depression, teens who have a sudden drop in grades, a sudden change in social activity, or moodiness beyond what you consider normal teen angst should talk to their social worker.

If you luck out, you may never have to deal with any of this. If you do, know that most teens with diabetes struggle. You are far from alone.

CHAPTER 19

Sick Day Management

Remember when a sick day for your child meant finding a warm blanket and a quiet activity, pushing some liquids and just letting them rest? All that changes with diabetes on board. Sick days for children with diabetes require more thought and care. This chapter will take you through several sick day situations from cuts and colds to broken bones and emergency room visits. With the proper preparation and forethought, you will be able to manage sick days with more ease.

Common Ailments and Diabetes

When is a cold not just a cold or an infection more than something that needs antibiotic cream? The answer is simple: when diabetes is present. While parents need not panic at the thought of an unrelated diabetes illness, they will need to take special care during those times, and understand the nuances of caring for a sick child with diabetes.

Head Colds and Viruses

Just because your child has the sniffles does not mean you have to dash to the emergency room. But when your child does battle minor ailments like a cold or mild virus, remember that her body is working extra hard and that means insulin needs can change. Any time your child is battling illness, be more vigilant.

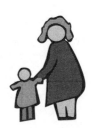

Check more often; think more carefully about boluses. The old wives' tale is that children always run higher when they are ill, but the truth is (like everything else in diabetes) each child's body reacts differently. Some run lower, some run higher, and a few lucky ones don't see any difference at all. Which is your child? You'll learn with time and experience.

If your child is ill enough to stay home from school or from playing with friends, it's not a bad idea to check her blood sugar every hour or so as long as the illness sticks around. In most cases, if your child is resting anyway, she won't mind too much. Even if she does, explain that while she is sick, you need to make extra sure she's okay. As the hours go by and things look fine and you realize it's just a cold, you can back off.

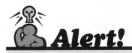

Alert!

Just because your child's blood sugars don't seem to fluctuate with his first few illnesses, don't begin to take that for granted. Always check extra on sick days, no matter what pattern you've seen.

Strep and Other Infections

If your child is spiking a fever, complaining of a sore throat, or is just completely wiped out, call your pediatrician (as you would with any child). If your pediatrician diagnoses some kind of infection, check in with your medical team and refer to the sick day plan they should have given you during diabetes training.

Even a sick day plan is simply a foundation and never the entire picture, because each illness might affect your child differently. The time of year could factor in (heat can sometimes mess with blood sugars) and the length of the illness. Don't feel funny calling your team if your child is ill enough to cause you concern. They are there to guide you through such things.

When you call, your team will most likely set up a different insulin dose schedule, at least for the next half day and ask you to check in again if you still have concerns. Sometimes, they may just tell you to watch your child closely, do regular checks, and see how things progress.

Essential

Ketones must be checked at least every four hours during any illness. Do not let in-range blood sugars stop you from doing this, because ketones can develop during illness at any time. The sooner you spot them, the better you can react.

As you watch your child through the illness, you'll begin to notice patterns. If your child is running higher than usual, you'll want to decide (with your team at first) how much more insulin to give and for how long. You'll also want to up your child's target range to give some padding in case the extra insulin ends up being too much.

If your child runs low, you'll need to work with your team to lower doses, and keep your child sipping something with carbs in it.

If your child's sore throat is keeping her from eating, use a sports drink, soda, juice, or even ice cream to keep her carb intake up. It's not always fun forcing your child to sip or eat when she just doesn't feel like it, but you need to find a way.

Cuts, Scrapes, and Breaks

What about cuts and infections? Despite the old myth that any cut or break is a crisis for a person with diabetes, you really can deal with them for the most part in a calm and almost nondiabetes manner.

Cuts and Scrapes

It is true that you need to be extra careful with cuts, particularly on your child's feet, but the perception that foot infection is a huge risk is really only for people whose diabetes is out of control for an extended period. Still, it's best to be aggressive in both avoiding and treating cuts, particularly on the feet. Treat a scrape or cut with a topical antibiotic and cover it. Watch it closely.

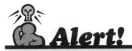

Alert!

As much as you want your child to be barefoot and carefree, encourage him to be sandal-footed and carefree instead. Avoiding scrapes, splinters, and other cuts on the bottom of the feet is the best defense against possible infections.

If a scrape or cut hangs around for a while, don't let it bother you. But if redness begins to show around the cut or spreads out from it, call your pediatrician. Your child may have developed an infection that requires antibiotics. As always, when in doubt, err on the side of caution. A phone call and a quick look by a doctor won't hurt and may be well worth the effort.

Breaks

Breaks are breaks, but the trauma may cause your child's blood sugars to act erratically. The healing body works hard and can use insulin at a quicker pace. As always in unusual situations, check your child's blood sugars more often and watch him closely.

If you do head to the doctor with a suspected broken bone, be sure to bring plenty of diabetes supplies, including extra sites and/or syringes, insulin, test strips, and ketone testing materials, just in case he is admitted to the hospital or worse, needs surgery.

If you are in a crisis, call a friend and ask her to run to your house and pick up your emergency pack. How to stock a sick day cabinet is presented later in the chapter.

There is no evidence that breaks heal more slowly for a person with diabetes. Expect your child's healing time to be the same as any child's. Check in with your medical team and let them know what has happened. Ask them if they want you to take any special precautions during the healing time, such as more frequent blood checks or daily ketone checks.

Stomach Bugs and Treatment

Then there's the Achilles' heel for some kids with diabetes: the stomach bug. It's hard to avoid them, and they always seem to come in seasons. Knowing how to react and when to call for help is a must when dealing with diabetes.

Signs a Bug Is Coming On

Your child has thrown up more than once and, you can tell, is well on her way to a third time. She may begin to spike a fever and looks lethargic and just plain ill. All these are signs that you may be in for a busy day with a stomach bug.

Often, you've heard that there is something going around school, or you know your child was at a birthday party where another child threw up. Don't ignore the signs. It's time to get busy. Stomach bugs can be the ultimate challenge in sick day management, and the sooner you can get ahead of them, the better off you are.

What to Do

First, try to keep your child ingesting at least some carbs on a regular basis. Even if it's just a spoonful of a soda or a sports drink every fifteen minutes, you're giving your child's body something to use with his insulin, and you're fighting to keep him hydrated; these are important goals as you battle this sickness. As a rule, try to get fifteen grams of carbohydrates per hour and up to one cup of fluid per hour into your child.

At the same time, never is it more crucial to check blood sugars and ketones then during a stomach illness. While some people's blood sugars soar, many have low blood sugars during vomiting bouts, particularly if they are on a peaking insulin such as NPH.

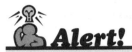

Alert!

Insulin can never be omitted. Even if your child does not feel like eating at all when he is sick, his body needs insulin, and you'll need to find a way to get carbs into him to match that insulin. Omitting insulin is a dangerous decision.

It's important to state this as many times as possible: Even if your child's blood sugars are within normal range, check constantly for ketones during a stomach illness. Use a ketone meter. The sooner you can detect ketones in the body, the easier it is to ward them off. Remember, as discussed in Chapter 6, the information gathered from ketone urine strips is at least two hours behind real time. Meters are up-to-the-minute, and your medical team will appreciate that information when you call them. Don't take in-range numbers for granted. Dehydration can cause ketones, and you won't want to wait until it's too late to find that out.

How can you tell if your child is holding anything down when she is throwing up? Generally speaking, if a liquid stays in her body for more than fifteen minutes, she is probably absorbing something. If her blood sugars remain above a number you and your endocrinologist are comfortable with, your child is probably ingesting at least a little bit of something.

As with any child with a stomach bug, stay away from dairy and stick to clear liquids. Some parents find that sugared Jell-O works well; it slides down the throat and into the belly without the child having to drink anything. Others like using a spoon and sugary liquid. It's up to you and your child. Do what works for you, as long as it works.

Time for More Help

If time ticks by and things are not getting better or, even worse, ketones are large and will not clear, it's time to get hands-on help. Sometimes, the only thing that will get a child with diabetes through a stomach bug is an IV with glucose and constant monitoring until ketones are cleared and he is eating and drinking again. If you feel overwhelmed or scared, push for your endocrinologist to have your child seen in the emergency room. It might be a few hours and it might be overnight. But the best thing is it will be a solution.

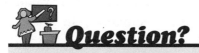 *Question?*

At what point should I call the medical team?
As soon as you know you are dealing with a stomach bug. You'll not only want their input, but you'll want to let them know you may need them in a moment's time at any time that day or night.

Emergency Room Visits

For some families, it never happens. For others, it's a common occurrence. But as a family with a child with diabetes, it's best to anticipate the possibility of an emergency room visit. As with most diabetes issues, being prepared is pivotal.

For Diabetes/Stomach Bug Issues

You've been talking to your endocrinologist, adjusting doses, forcing liquids down your child's throat, and he's still throwing up and spilling ketones. When is it time to call for help? Put simply: When you cannot handle it on your own anymore.

Sometimes, during stomach bugs, the best treatment for a child is an IV with glucose in it to match their insulin. Since most parents don't know how to do IVs at home (nor should they), if your child is spilling ketones and throwing up, your medical team will want to draw labs regularly to make sure he comes around to where he should be. So the hospital is the place to go.

It's important that your endocrinologist call the emergency room before you arrive. If possible, head to the emergency room that actually has a pediatric endocrinologist on staff. If you are far from one, have your team call before you get there and connect with a physician, so he or she is sure to consult your team in your child's care.

Of course, if it's a crisis, you'll need to go to the closest ER. But if you feel confident you can make it to the one your medical team is affiliated with, it's better.

When you arrive, you probably won't have to sit in a waiting room. Ketones (possibly DKA) or constant vomiting with ketones and a low blood sugar is a true emergency. If your endocrinologist has not made that clear, politely explain it to the triage folks. If you need to, ask them to call your medical team for reassurance.

When you get into the ER, your child will be immediately assessed to make sure he is not going into DKA and then to decide on a plan. In most cases with stomach bugs, time on an IV does the trick. Sometimes, if your child is prone to bugs, he might be admitted for twenty-four hours or asked to stay until he is eating, drinking, and not vomiting.

If it's DKA, expect to be admitted. This situation needs to be treated with the utmost care, since forcing a child's blood sugar back down too quickly can bring other complications.

What to Bring

When you leave for the ER you'll be in a rush, but try to bring a few things to make you and your child more comfortable. Dress in loose, comfortable clothing since you may be by your child's side for hours and hours. Bring along a favorite comfort item such as a blanket or stuffed animal for your child. Bring your cell phone, but turn it off inside the ER. Still, you'll want to be able to step outside and make calls to update friends and family if needed.

Nondiabetes ER Visits

If you have to head to the ER for a break or stitches or some other kind of emergency, you'll still want to let your endocrinologist know where you are heading and let the medical team know, right away, that your child has diabetes.

Unlike DKA or the stomach bug, your child doesn't need special treatment in the waiting room (and while it's tempting to use diabetes to cut to the front of the line, don't set this poor example for your child). Let the nurse at the check-in desk know that besides the injury at hand, your child does have Type 1 diabetes, and be sure to tell every person handling your child as well.

What about checking blood sugars while in the ER? Some parents are enraged when the staff insists on doing it by themselves on their equipment, but at times, hospital rules have to come first. Offer to do the checking yourself, and if they decline, be understanding. (You can always do your own checking for your own peace of mind while in there as well.) Let them know that, even though your child is being treated for a nondiabetes issue, you'll want to check more often than usual to make sure the stress is not playing games with blood sugars and ketones.

Stocking Your Sick Day Cabinet

As if enough drawers have not been taken over by diabetes supplies, you'll need to dedicate another cabinet, shelf, or drawer to the things you need to treat your child on sick days. A sick day cabinet or drawer means you'll be able to find all you need in one spot at a time when you may be too worried to have to search your home for an item.

Diabetes Tools

You already have your strips and meters and ketone-checking supplies and insulin in one place, so you don't need to double it up here. But you do need to pack a small bag with a few of each item. That way, if you need to rush out the door in an emergency, it's all there without your having to think through what to pack and bring.

Your cabinet should also have some other tools you'll need, including an eight-ounce measuring cup. This cup can be filled with the sugary liquid you choose to have your child drink during the sickness. You won't need to guess how much your child has ingested; you can just look at the cup and do the math. You'll also want to keep on hand some juice boxes, crackers, and other foods your child does not mind when she is sick. Don't count on them being in your cabinet, since in life, we all run out of everything.

 Essential

Make sure you let babysitters and all family members know where the sick day cabinet is and what it is for. If you are on the road and need to talk someone through something, it is better that they have a basic knowledge first to save time and stress.

You'll also want to tuck a list of your child's medical providers and their phone numbers in this cabinet, and a second one in your sick day bag. In a crisis, it's easy to forget a phone number even if you dial it all the time. How many times have you been asked a phone number only to think, "Gosh, I think it's speed-dial seven." Having the phone numbers on hand will help in an emergency.

It's also a good idea to tuck a blank logbook into your cabinet and bag. Even if you don't usually write down numbers, a sick day is one time you simply must. Having a logbook on hand will make that easier, and help your medical team have better information to help your child.

Medications for Other Illnesses

Talk to your medical team about what cold and cough medicines they recommend and how to use them. Some medications contain fructose, but your medical team may still like them better. Purchase those items and put them in the sick day cabinet, apart from the rest of the family's needs. You don't want to run out of the only medication you can use on your child with diabetes.

Also tuck in some antibiotic cream, bandages, and other supplies for cuts and scrapes your child may get. Good care means no infections.

Other Long-Term Health Issues

Diabetes can be complicated by the presence of other long-term illnesses, and if one does pop up, you and your medical team will need to regroup to carefully plan how to deal with it. Some of these illnesses are more common to kids with diabetes and others are not. All need extra care.

Thyroid Issues

It is estimated that at least one in every ten children with diabetes will develop either hypothyroidism (an underactive thyroid gland) or hyperthyroidism (an overactive thyroid gland). Your medical team should be feeling your child's thyroid and running a screening for thyroid antibodies on a regular basis. Usually, with vigilant watch, a child's thyroid disease can be caught and treated with medications early on, since medical teams tend to look closely for this issue.

If your child is diagnosed with a thyroid disease, you may feel devastated that your child has yet another issue to deal with. But in reality, dealing with thyroid disease is simple compared to diabetes. Most children take one pill a day and have labs drawn (at the same time as their diabetes labs) to make sure the dosage is correct. Beyond that, there is little daily impact on a child's life.

Usually, once a child is on medication, the thyroid issue does not affect daily living or blood sugars. A symptom of an underactive thyroid gland is weight gain, and for overactive, it is weight loss. If you see a sudden change either way, call your endocrinologist and talk about the possibility of thyroid issues in your child.

Celiac Disease

The name strikes fear into the hearts of all diabetes parents. Celiac disease, in which the body cannot process glutens, a protein found in wheat and other grains, is more common in children with diabetes than in children without. Although the chances are rare, you should insist your child be tested for celiac disease at least every two years.

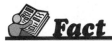 **Fact**

> According to the American Diabetes Association, about one in twenty people with diabetes also have celiac disease. Your medical team should regularly check your child for celiac disease. If they don't, ask the team for an explanation you can understand.

Children with diabetes who develop celiac face a double whammy: Not only do they need to count every carb they eat and give insulin for it because of the diabetes, they also have to severely limit what types of food they eat because of celiac disease. Some parents find their children's blood sugars fluctuate when celiac is not treated right. When a child with celiac eats gluten, the lining of the small intestine suffers damage and the child has trouble eating. Your team should work with you and your child to find a diet acceptable to her so she can live with both diseases.

CHAPTER 20

Advocacy and Fundraising: Are They Right for You?

There's a whole world of advocacy and fundraising groups working to make living with diabetes better and, ultimately, to cure the disease. Whether you and your family join that world is a personal decision, one that includes what you think you'd do best and whom you'd like to join. This chapter will introduce you to some of the more prominent groups in diabetes circles and also help you explore if volunteering or fundraising is right for you.

The Advocacy and Fundraising World

Even just three decades ago, people with diabetes weren't organized to move toward a better future, and because there were few good treatment options for diabetes, many kept their disease a secret. Thanks to the work of parents of kids with diabetes and people with diabetes, however, now there are more options. Before deciding where to volunteer, it's important to know what advocacy and fundraising can mean.

Advocacy

Advocacy in diabetes comes in two types: advocating for issues like patient rights and treatments, and advocating for Congress to vote for bills and funding that will help diabetes research move forward. The first type of advocacy usually is in the form of support groups, online programs, and outreach programs that you'd join to help other families new to diabetes.

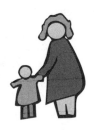

Advocacy to encourage Congress to be more supportive of diabetes needs is more about getting your voice heard. Although you may be uncomfortable storming Capitol Hill, it does not have to be that intense.

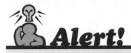
Alert!

If you want to advocate, lend your voice to an established group. There are excellent options when it comes to choosing a strong and proven group, so don't try to reinvent the wheel. Your voice will be louder as part of a recognized and respected team.

Most advocacy groups are constantly building their troops in the field. You can sign on via e-mail to receive alerts that keep you apprised of what is going on in terms of diabetes legislation on Capitol Hill and what you can do. Sometimes, you'll be asked to send a letter or make a phone call. If you'd like, you can even visit legislators to get your point across. Few things are more empowering to a parent than being heard, first person, by his or her nation's leaders. Grass-roots advocacy can help you do just that.

Fundraising

Okay, so you feel funny about it: How can you ask your friends to give you their hard-earned money? The truth is that most friends wish they could find a way to help you, and in the world of kids and diabetes, there are not many options. Asking friends to sign on to walk for your child or to make a donation to a diabetes charity you support may just be the perfect way to help them feel empowered.

Fundraising can also give your child hope. More than a few children, after attending their first Walk to Cure Diabetes event, have told their parents they could just feel a cure in their future. As hard as she has to work every day to stay healthy, a walk or another type of fundraiser reminds your child that the world cares. So how does a family choose an organization to put their advocacy and/or fundraising time behind? It's all about the mission, and it's also about personal choice. Do know, as you decide, that every reputable group in our nation is doing a good job for our kids. As long as it's a well-run organization, you've made the right choice.

The American Diabetes Association (ADA)

Founded in 1940, the American Diabetes Association has a mission, to this day, to help people with both Type 1 and Type 2 diabetes. The ADA's work runs the gamut, everything from funding research for both diseases to conducting educational programs.

How They Operate

Although the ADA does fund research, most of its efforts are based on education, support, and daily living with diabetes. The ADA's main focus is building a better world for people living with the disease and educating those who help people with diabetes.

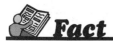

Fact

In 2005, the American Diabetes Association funded $40 million in research for diabetes, split between Type 1 and Type 2 issues, and some encompassing both. That funding came out of the $132 million raised that year, with the majority going to educational programs.

Many parents are drawn to the ADA at the start because of its many educational programs. The ADA holds the largest diabetes gathering in the nation each June at a select location, with close to 20,000 people attending scientific sessions, educational programs, and advocacy events. ADA also has a close relationship with Certified Diabetes Educators and pediatric endocrinologists, since many are part of their organization for educational reasons.

As part of the ADA, you'll be working to help Type 1 and Type 2 diabetes, rather than focusing on Type 1. Again, this is a personal decision. The ADA has chapters across the nation that can be found by logging onto *www.diabetes.org*.

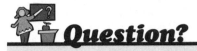

Question?

Does the ADA support Type 1 families?
Absolutely. The educational programs help families with daily care and school issues, and the ADA is also a great supporter of diabetes camps.

The ADA's main fundraising events include a national Walk For Diabetes, the Tour de Cure bike-a-thon held in many spots around the country, and the new "Kiss a Pig" fundraiser that's a humorous tweak at thanking the pig for its part in diabetes research. Pig islets were long used to make insulin, and now, pig islets are being experimented with for possible xenotransplantation, or placing them into human bodies to replace damaged human islet cells.

The ADA and Advocacy

The ADA has an active advocacy program, asking its members to contact Congress and local officials about bills and issues that affect people with diabetes. The variety of issues is wide, since they focus on Type 1, Type 2, and government advocacy as well. The biannual "Call to Congress" invites adults and children alike to visit elected officials on Capitol Hill to talk about diabetes and what the government can do. The ADA often asks advocates to be vocal about bills on the hill and even some state issues.

The Juvenile Diabetes Research Foundation (JDRF)

Founded in 1970 by two sets of parents of children with diabetes who were sitting at a kitchen table lamenting the lack of support and research focused solely on Type 1 diabetes, the JDRF is now the nation's top non-governmental supporter of diabetes research of all kinds.

What the JDRF Does Best

The JDRF's mission is very clear: to find a cure for diabetes and its complications through the support of research. While JDRF has educational and outreach programs, the absolute main focus is research for a cure for diabetes and its complications. The organization works hard to help people on a daily basis who are struggling with Type 1 diabetes, but it is unabashed in its dedication to funding research for a cure.

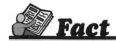 **Fact**

In 2005, JDRF funded more than $123 million in research for a cure for diabetes and its complications. The total budget that year was $186 million, meaning the vast majority of the work is aimed at a cure.

The JDRF has held support groups and "networking coffees" for parents and kids dealing with Type 1 diabetes for years, but three years ago, the organization jumped deeper into the outreach and support category by introducing the Online Diabetes Support Team (ODST), a group of cyber volunteers who can help anyone dealing with diabetes anywhere and at any time of day. The average response time for someone logging on and asking the ODST for help is less than one day.

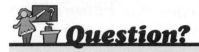

Question?

Does the JDRF do anything for Type 2?
Yes. Because more than $36 million of the research funded by the JDRF studies complications, the Type 2 community benefits from this work as well.

The JDRF also has a signature outreach program called the Bag of Hope. A bag of diabetes goodies, including books, videos, tools, and Rufus the Teddy Bear with Diabetes, is delivered to new families. Like a Welcome Wagon for diabetes, the best part of the Bag of Hope is the volunteer who gets it to you: usually another parent dealing with exactly what you are dealing with.

The JDRF has four main areas of fundraising: the JDRF Walk to Cure Diabetes, a national event spread over the year that's one of the top fundraising walks in any kind of charity group; the special events such as galas and golf tournaments held in cities across the nation annually; the major gifts program; and the new Ride to Cure Diabetes, a 100-mile ride held in a number of spots, including Death Valley. The JDRF expects to cross the $200 million level in annual funds raised in 2007. In total, as of 2006, it has funded more than $900 million in diabetes research since their inception.

The JDRF and Advocacy

When it comes to advocacy, the JDRF is a powerhouse. In 2004, the *Wall Street Journal* wrote of the JDRF advocacy program, "Not since AIDS activists stormed scientific meetings in the 1980s has a patient group done more to set the agenda of medical research." The JDRF's advocates number nearly 40,000 and take on issues via e-mail, phone calls, and visits to local offices and even Capitol Hill.

Two of the JDRF's premier events include the Promise to Remember Me campaign, held every other year, when kids with diabetes visit their U.S. senators and congressional representatives at their district offices and ask them to remember to help cure diabetes, and the biannual JDRF Children's Congress, which chooses 150 children from across the nation to visit Capitol Hill and lobby for a cure. Information on both programs can be found at the JDRF Web site.

Other Big Names

While the ADA and the JDRF are the big boys on the block, there are some other movers and shakers out there that could use your help. Some parents like the smaller groups; others choose to support the big guys and some smaller ones.

Children with Diabetes

The father of a little girl with diabetes started Children with Diabetes as a Web site. What founder Jeff Hitchcock was hoping to create was a Web site where his young daughter could meet other kids with diabetes. What he ended up with was *www.childrenwith diabetes.com*, one of the most respected and used online forums. Hitchcock's formula was part brilliance and part timing: When he launched CWD in 1995, the notion of online support was very much in its infancy.

The Web site grew with the industry, becoming sleeker and stocked with vital information and taking on advertising. Eventually, it became a live program as well, with regional conferences and the Friends for Life Conference held each year and drawing in more than 2,000 families with children with diabetes.

Spreading into funding as well, CWD's charitable foundation has helped support the International Diabetes Youth Foundation (IDYA) and has given about $50,000 to other diabetes charities. But support is the main thing CWD does, and its volunteers are focused on that. Does it work? Consider this: The Web site averages 15,000 hits *per day.*

The Diabetes Research Institute (DRI)

Based in Miami, the DRI might be small, but it packs a big punch. Led by scientific director Dr. Camillo Ricordi, the DRI has been near the front of many diabetes research breakthroughs, including islet cell transplantation and pancreatic stem cell development. While a good chunk of its funding comes from groups such as the JDRF, the DRI raises some of its own money as well. The institute has been credited with a good part of many diabetes milestones, such as the landmark 1978 study that led to better pregnancy results for women with Type 1 diabetes. The DRI has supporters around the world and holds research briefings in New York City as well as other locations.

Is Volunteering Right for You?

Although the common belief is that anyone touched by diabetes should help push toward a cure, not everyone is up for it. Figuring out if you are and how you fit into the big picture will help make the experience positive all the way around.

Good Points to Ponder

Many parents and caregivers find reaching out and volunteering is a great way to surround themselves with people who know their plight and care about what is going on. No matter what organization you choose, you'll be entering a world where you don't have to translate medical jargon or explain what a high or low blood sugar is. That's a big benefit to volunteering, and one that makes it almost worth the while on its own.

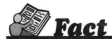 **Fact**

A study by the Points of Light Foundation found that children of parents who volunteer find they have more respect for their parents and believe their parents care about the community.

But you can get much more than that. Caring for a child with diabetes can, at times, defeat you. There is no remission, no time when you can say, "There, I've fixed her." For parents and caregivers, that feeling of treading water can be depressing. In volunteering, you can find a way to feel as though you're making progress.

Volunteering can show your child that you are doing all you can to help her reach a point where she can live diabetes-free. Not only can you win the respect of your child from doing good, you can remind her, when the chips are down, that you're doing everything you can to help her be cured.

Timing Is Everything

So diving in to volunteer can be a good choice for parents. It's a good idea, though, to think about the timing. Some caregivers are ready and willing from the day their child is diagnosed; more need a little time to get used to life with diabetes before taking on additional responsibilities. You don't want to commit yourself before you've moved somewhat past the initial process of grief and anger; nor do you want to let your volunteer work supersede your job as the parent of a child with diabetes.

 Essential

A good rule for when to engage in volunteer activities is the "one-year cycle." Once you've been through a full year since diagnosis and faced every holiday and special event like back to school and parties, you're ready to take the next step.

If you think you've got your feet on the ground and you're coping with the day-to-day challenges of diabetes, consider volunteering. Once you've chosen the group with the mission that best suits you, call the local office and ask how you can help.

Start Out Slowly

By starting out with a short, easy role, you can make sure you like the people and agree with the mission. In time, when and if you do agree, you can decide where you want to go in the group. At that time, treat it like a job: Talk to the leaders about how you think you'd fit and the "volunteer career path" you'd like to take. Don't be shy; the organization, if it's a good one, will want to match your expectations and desires.

Don't be afraid to try something new when volunteering. If you work in the media, the organization may naturally want to put you on PR assignments. That's fine if it's what you want. But if you've always wanted to try your hand at government relations or finances or fundraising, speak up. You are a valuable commodity and any good organization will work with you to match your skills with a job or jobs that intrigue you.

Good for Your Child?

Think of your children when jumping into volunteer opportunities as well because the situation can be both a help and a hindrance for them. Younger children, for the most part, get a big kick out of volunteering. For fundraisers like walks and galas, younger kids love the attention and party-like atmosphere. For advocacy issues, younger kids find visiting big-name politicians "cool" and interesting. For the most part, little kids are easy to bring along on any of these types of events.

As kids get older, it will be important to have their buy-in on anything you ask them to do and even anything you do in their name. It's their disease and their life, and while you as a parent want to do all you can to change their future, you need to consider their present life too.

 Essential

When you look at getting involved, be sure to talk to your child about the benefits, not just long term (in other words, a cure) but short term, for him. Talk about community service hours and life experiences as well.

Older kids will be thinking about their college applications and community service hours for school and graduation. It's natural to suggest they take part in diabetes programs to gain an advantage in these areas, but make sure they don't mind. Some teens want to have one part of their life that has nothing to do with diabetes. If this describes your child, respect that and discuss what she is comfortable with you doing even if she chooses to step aside.

In every way you can, encourage your child to reap some benefits from his situation. Advocacy work can lead to an insider view of Washington and politics and can help a child build a network that comes in handy when it's time to apply to college. Fundraising events can be like parties for kids; a time to get together with all kinds of friends.

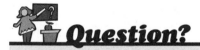 **Question?**

Can we celebrate diagnosis day?
Absolutely. A giant party/fundraiser each year around diagnosis day can be like another birthday, and a time for everyone to say to your child, "Good job this year." Start the tradition now.

Involvement can also give your child something more powerful than experience and connections: It can give them hope. A child who sees firsthand that thousands of people are working to cure them knows deep down that the world truly cares—and that's worth every hour of volunteering you can add up.

When It's Wrong

Some rare times, volunteering for fundraising and advocacy isn't the right choice. Families and parents need to be careful if this is the case and not push a child into a situation she does not want.

Poster Child Syndrome

Some children start out gung ho, always willing to speak in pub-lic and meet with others about diabetes and the need for a cure. Then, in time, they begin to feel as if they aren't living up to what they should be. This is called the "poster child syndrome," and in the case of a very involved family, it needs to be treated with care.

If your child has been held up as an example of a child who always does the right thing with her diabetes, it's more difficult for her when she slips (and most children do occasionally slip in their care). She might be afraid to let anyone down, and she might keep her struggle with diabetes a secret until it is dangerously late. If your child is a public face in the diabetes world, encourage her to be honest from the start. Don't let her say she's always perfect; make her understand that diabetes is hard, and that's why you're trying to cure it.

Needing Separation

Other children can feel as though diabetes takes over their lives if it's what they have to do even in their downtime. If your child com-plains, ask her if there are events she likes and ones she doesn't. Come up with a compromise that works for her and for you, so you can keep your family working toward a cure and not burn your child out.

Parent Burnout

It's not easy as a parent to burn out on diabetes advocacy. After all, you know your children never get a moment off from diabetes. So how can you look yourself in the eye if you burn out? But par-ents have to pace themselves as well. Although you want to give all you can, if you get to a point where you feel you just need to step back, you absolutely should. Sometimes, a breather gives a person just what he needs to become re-energized and renew the fight that most parents can never say they're done with—the fight to cure their child.

CHAPTER 21

The Path to a Bright Future

A fter the invention of insulin in the late 1920s, not much happened to advance diabetes treatment or find a cure for decades. Over the past fifteen years, however, better, more humane therapies have become available. There is hope, in the not-too-distant future, for a cure. There is hope that parents and care-givers of children with diabetes will be able to embrace a future, in which, with their help, diabetes will be a distant memory.

Twenty-five Years Ago

The year 1980 doesn't sound so long ago, but in diabetes care, it is another generation. Although many parents of children with diabetes were adults by that time (and we still feel young), we have truly progressed a lifetime in diabetes care since that time.

Insulin Options

Just a short time ago, parents had little choice of how to treat their child's diabetes on a daily basis. For the most part, children were on one or perhaps two shots a day of a peaking, middle-acting insulin like NPH. Some children took regular-acting insulin as well, which had to be administered exactly a half hour before eating and peaked twice in a six-hour period.

The scenes in the 1989 film *Steel Magnolias*, with Sally Field and Julia Roberts, that captured the world of diabetes, were all too real. With little understanding of how to better use insulin to work with food, lows could come crashing down on a person with diabetes with little warning, as seen in Julia's character just before her wedding day.

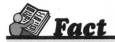 **Fact**

> Even disposable needles were a new notion just a few years ago. Most children had to reuse a large, painful needle that had to be boiled for sanitation and then sharpened in order to be used. These needles caused unsightly scar tissue to build up on small bodies.

Some astute endocrinologists and families figured out that eating more often and at scheduled times, as well as taking shots more frequently, would help "control" diabetes to a point. But for the most part, it was a matter of injecting insulin and crossing your fingers. Those were still the days of "brittle" diabetes, and there was little hope for a better future.

Past Tools

Glucose meters had come to market by then, but they were not covered by insurance, and they were bulky and difficult to use. Most families did not have access to meters because they were too expensive and depended on lab-drawn blood sugar readings and urine dips to figure out what was going on with their child's diabetes.

These tests were random at best and gave families little information on which to base decisions. Checking a person's blood sugar multiple times throughout the day was barely considered, and other than knowing their child was high or low, many families knew little of the moment-to-moment changes in their child's blood sugar levels.

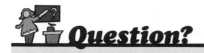

Question?

Families, up until the early 1990s, for the most part relied on tablets dropped in urine. Each tablet would produce a color, depending on how much glucose was in the urine. It was a rough tool based on old information, and hard for parents to use to make any real decisions.

Pumps were a rarity, too, although they premiered in 1980. In this decade, the notion of adults, never mind children, on pumps was seldom discussed. It was not until the 1990s and even the start of the twenty-first century that children on pumps became the norm.

Better Treatment Options Are Here

That is now officially history. Parents and caregivers have many options; with education, research, and hard work, they can find the newest and smartest ways to keep their children healthy until a cure is found.

Insulin Options

As discussed in Chapter 6, new insulin options are available today, and by keeping a close eye on the industry, parents can stay ahead of what is coming out in the near future. No longer does a family need to settle for a set meal plan and set times for shots and snacks. Rather, you can sit down with your medical team, look at the almost endless choices of insulin, and find those that work best with the lifestyle you'd like your child to have.

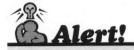

Alert!

Every insulin acts a tiny bit differently in each child. While it's great to take advice from frlends with children on other insulin choices, make sure you work with your medical team to figure out if it's the right choice for your child.

Some doctors are also experimenting with other drugs that interact better with insulin, such as pills that are usually used for Type 2 diabetes that can help people with Type 1 better use their insulin. There is also a drug called Symlin that some diabetes patients inject to help level out their blood sugars, particularly just after meals. The idea of a second drug that makes insulin work better is leading some endocrinologists to wonder if A1cs constantly in the 6s, until now almost an impossible task, could be achieved more easily in the near future.

Better Pumps

Pump companies, now fueled by a hungry market, are also working to create better products. As discussed in Chapter 6, not long ago there were only two or three choices. Today, there are more than eight kinds of pumps, and more are coming to market soon. Some companies are even offering upgrade programs that allow you to upgrade to the newest model for a reasonable price; these programs keep you up-to-date in pump care instead of having to hold on to an older model until its warranty expires and insurance helps you again.

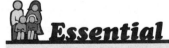

Essential

The best place to stay current on pump technology is the nonprofit site, *www.insulin-pumpers.org*. The site has descriptions, reviews, and all the latest information on all pump models; there are also regular chat sessions with pump company staffers.

Look for pumps today to interact with your personal computer, make bolus suggestions, keep track of "insulin on board," and even marry to meters. Most, if not all, are now water-resistant, and most are durable enough and portable enough to be usable on children of any age.

The Artificial Pancreas

The Holy Grail of pump therapy, if you will, will be the advent of the artificial pancreas, something that has become truly foreseeable since 2005. With patient groups pushing and researchers wanting this to happen, it now seems closer to reality than ever.

The artificial pancreas is not a new concept. The smart pump or artificial pancreas would constantly track blood sugars and react using an algorithm to give insulin as the body needs it, but it's been something few could get their hands around. Researchers and scientists have struggled with how to make it happen, and with little public support, they had little motivation.

Then, in 2005, the Juvenile Diabetes Research Foundation was approached by a volunteer who wanted to see that change. Frustrated with waiting for the true cure, the parent offered a million dollars for the JDRF to look into pushing forward an artificial pancreas. It worked. Months later, the JDRF's Artificial Pancreas Project was born. The project's short-term goal is to deliver to market a continuous sensor that not only works well for adults and kids alike but is covered by insurance and available to everyone. The longer-term goal is to marry that sensor to a pump and have them interact and work independently from the person, and, eventually, become one item that works as a pancreas, keeping blood sugars level on a constant basis.

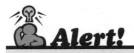

Alert!

For up-to-date information on the Artificial Pancreas Project, log onto ✐*www.jdrf.org* and sign up for the Artificial Pancreas Project newsletter. You'll get updates via e-mail as the project progresses.

The JDRF has helped spur lots of activity in this area and has set a goal of pushing to make it happen sooner than it ever would have without their support and the support of the tens of thousands of families they represent.

Continuous Sensors

Some children across the nation are on continuous sensors now, either as part of a clinical trial or with their parents paying for them. The early statistics are good: People on these sensors seem to experience an almost immediate (a few weeks) drop in A1cs. They are also finding that food and insulin do things in their bodies they never realized before. Think of it this way: Even with ten or more blood checks a day, you are only finding out what your child's blood sugar is a tiny fraction of the time. With a continuous sensor, you have almost to-the-moment information and can spot trends such as post-meal spikes that you can then attack better.

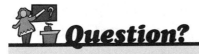

Question?

Is the continuous sensor right for my child now?
That's a personal question, and one that your child needs to help answer. It's not easy to wear and run a second device. Make sure your child is on board before you investigate the possibility, as tempting as it is.

The Artificial Pancreas Project (APP) is receiving lots of buzz, with articles in many major publications, and it is helping families remain hopeful for better daily care as they continue to work for and watch for the biological cure.

Cures on the Horizon

As exciting as the notion of an artificial pancreas is, parents and caregivers are not giving up on a true biological cure for diabetes, either through islet cell replacement or regeneration. Work continues to progress, and hope is there as well.

Islet Cell Replacement

The buzz was huge in 2000 when the Edmonton Protocol was announced. Cadaver islet cells were used to replace the destroyed cells in a group of patients with Type 1 diabetes. With the help of some strong immunosuppressant drugs, the patients were able to remain insulin-free, some for more than five years. At the time, it was hailed as a near cure, a possible end to the question of how diabetes would be cured.

But some concerns lingered. The drugs given to keep the autoimmunity from attacking the new working islets were harsh; children could never go on them. Only patients in dire straits were considered. Most of the patients were eventually (within two to five years) back on insulin. In time, the scientific community realized that this procedure was not the "cure," but it was a breakthrough.

Although most patients eventually ended up back on insulin, they also regained their ability to feel lows coming on; most of them had lost this ability, which had led to difficulty living their normal lives. Also, the procedure showed that islets can be easily "transplanted" into the body with just a day-patient treatment. All this data will help scientists move forward in search of a true cure.

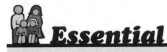 **Essential**

Learning about the Edmonton Protocol is as easy as going to ✍www .diabetes123.com, clicking on the News and Information link and then clicking on The Edmonton Protocol for Islet Transplants. It's worth understanding it in its entirety.

Regeneration of Islets

Scientists have also discovered something intriguing: Even in patients who have had diabetes for more than two decades, a tiny bit of islet cell activity remains. That finding brought forth the concept of islet cell regeneration. If researchers could coax the body's remaining cells into creating new cells, the body could replace its dying cells on its own, eliminating the need for any kind of transplant. In other words, the patient would no longer need any kind of immunosuppressant drugs, since the replacement cells would come from their own body. Researchers around the world are working on this concept daily. Regeneration could also eliminate the need for a large amount of islet cells from cadavers or another source, something that scientists are struggling with now as well.

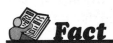 **Fact**

If scientists can find a way to get a human body to constantly reproduce islet cells, they could find a way for the body to fight off autoimmune diabetes for good.

Regeneration is still being studied in animal models, but groups like the Diabetes Research Institute and the Juvenile Diabetes Research Foundation are dedicating millions of dollars to push the science forward.

Stopping Autoimmunity

Drugs, such as AntiCD-3, are in human clinical trial right now to reverse autoimmunity in people with diabetes, as well as with other autoimmune diseases such as celiac disease and psoriasis. If these drugs work well in humans, they could, when combined with regeneration or islet cell replacement, bring researchers closer to the entire puzzle of a cure for diabetes. They could also be used to stop the progression of diabetes when detected early, protecting the remaining functioning islet cells before too many are killed off and, thus, stopping the onset of Type 1 before a child is fully diagnosed.

Complications

It used to be a given that if you battled diabetes for long enough, you'd suffer the complications: kidney disease, blindness, heart ailments, and even amputations. But today, better care and proactive work against those threats have changed the future.

Kidney Disease

The kidneys were once and still are one of the prime targets of diabetes complications. Many if not most people suffering with diabetes eventually faced the need for dialysis and, eventually, the need for a transplant. But today, frequent lab tests that monitor kidney function and proactive treatment when any kind of early trouble is detected have cut the stats on kidney disease and diabetes.

The Diabetes Control and Complications Trial (DCCT), a nine-year study by the National Institutes of Health, showed that tight control of blood glucose levels reduced the chance of kidney disease in people with diabetes by 50 percent. Before the DCCT, it was thought that kidney disease was inevitable. Now, people understand they can help offset kidney disease and even avoid it, although it involves a lot of hard work to do so. (See Chapter 6 for more information on the DCCT.)

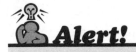

Alert!

Ask your medical team how often they do labs to check your child's kidney functions. Insist on having the labs drawn once a year, even if your child is in the early years of diagnosis or is showing no signs of kidney trouble.

Since the mid-1990s, many doctors have begun treating patients with a type of medication called ACE Inhibitors the moment they begin to spill protein into urine (an early sign of kidney distress). ACE Inhibitors, used to treat hypertension, have proven to slow down and even avoid the onset of kidney disease by nearly 50 percent in people who showed first signs of progression to the disease. The use of ACE inhibitors is slowing the rates of kidney disease in people with diabetes even more.

Eye Issues

Blindness was once thought to be an inevitable complication for many people battling diabetes. High levels of blood glucose attack the extremities first, and the capillaries in the eyes are often the first to be damaged. But again, the DCCT showed that tight control offsets this complication and often removed it completely.

Doctors also have improved methods of looking at eyes and keeping ahead of diabetes troubles; they are now able to use laser surgery to correct what would once have led to blindness. With a good ophthalmologist who specializes in diabetes checking your child annually, you should be able to ensure that this complication will never attack your child as well.

Amputations and Other Fears

Again, tight control and better tools mean that statistics for today's generation will be much different than in the past. With better pumps, insulin, and other drugs to help insulin work, even doctors are not sure what the future will hold, but they do know that the statistics will just keep getting better and better.

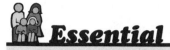
Essential

> If your child hears horror stories of amputations and the like, tell her with all confidence that that was a different time. Today's technology has changed her future to one that is bright and filled with hope.

Parents should discuss complications in a private meeting with their child's medical team. Your team should give you confidence in the future and an understanding of their plan of attack to stay ahead of any diabetes-related complications so that they play no part in your child's future.

What You Can Do

The future is indeed bright, but that does not mean diabetes patients don't have to work hard. Maintaining tight control and battling highs and lows is hard work that weighs heavily on a child and his family over the years. That's why, in the end, a biological cure is the real answer. Every family needs to work hard but not give up on that goal. Once they settle into life with diabetes, every family must ask themselves every day: Am I doing all I can to help reach the goal of a biological cure?

Fundraising

As discussed in Chapter 20, there are plenty of places that need your help financially. You don't have to be a millionaire to make a difference. With close to one million people suffering from Type 1 diabetes in America, if each person gave $100 a year, a billion dollars a year would flow into research for better care and a cure. Find a way that you can pitch in. Form a walk team. Write a check. Ask your boss to match it. There's power in numbers, and every family just needs to pitch in a bit to achieve the goal.

Speaking Out

The same goes for your voice. It takes time to settle into this life with diabetes, but once you do, never settle for it for your child. Educate yourself by reading all the updated diabetes information you can.

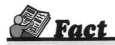

Google can send you a daily update on diabetes issues. Log onto google.com and sign up for a daily list of articles that discuss Type 1 diabetes; you'll have a record of everything new going on in the field, as well as new advancements, recent findings, and study results.

Find a place that you know will help you learn and understand. Then find a way to speak out. Sign on as a diabetes advocate with the Juvenile Diabetes Research Foundation. Write letters and e-mail your elected officials to let them know you are watching how they vote on important issues such as funding for the National Institutes of Health. As part of a large team of voices, you will be heard.

In the end, no book or treatment or understanding of daily care will ever add up to what a cure will mean: freedom for your child, for your family, and for you from the burden of diabetes.

That's a solution that needs no subtext.

Glossary

A1c test—A lab-drawn test that shows the three-month average of blood sugars.

ACE Inhibitors—A type of drug used to lower blood pressure. Studies indicated it may prevent or slow the progression of kidney disease in people with diabetes.

Adult-onset diabetes—Now known as Type 2 diabetes, in this type of diabetes the body still produces insulin but has trouble using it. It can be controlled by diet and exercise.

Advocacy—Speaking out and pushing for changes in government, in schools, and throughout the world.

American Diabetes Association (ADA)—National group that raises money and awareness for Type 1 and Type 2 diabetes; Web site: ☞ www.diabetes.org.

Antibody—A large Y-shaped protein used by the immune system to identify and neutralize foreign objects like bacteria and viruses. In diabetes, antibodies get confused and attack the beta cells rather than protecting them.

Autoimmune diabetes—Another name for Type 1 diabetes; the body destroys its own islet-producing cells and loses the ability to produce insulin.

Autoimmunity—The immune response an organism launches against its own cells or tissues.

Basal rates—A continuous twenty-four-hour set pattern of insulin delivery, usually on an insulin pump; also called background insulin.

Beta cells—Insulin-producing cells in the pancreas.

Blood glucose—The main sugar that the body makes from food, and the main source of energy for cells; it is carried through the bloodstream.

Blood glucose level—The concentration of glucose in the blood, measured in milligrams per deciliter in the United States.

Blood glucose meter—A hand-held machine that uses a drop of blood to measure blood glucose level in a person.

Blood sugar—The level of glucose in the blood as measured by lab test or on a meter.

Bolus—An amount of insulin given at one time either to lower blood sugar or to cover the carbs consumed at a meal.

Carb bolus—An amount of insulin given to match the food eaten.

Carbohydrates, or carbs—One of the main constituents of food; composed mainly of sugar and starches.

Carb ratio—The equation that determines how much insulin is needed per gram of carbohydrates. For instance, an average carb ratio is 1 unit of insulin to 15 grams of carb.

Cannula—The short tubing inserted into the body as part of a pump site; attached to tubing, it delivers insulin to the body from the pump.

Certified Diabetes Educator (CDE)—A health care professional certified by the

American Association of Diabetes Educators to teach people how to manage diabetes.

C-peptide—A by-product of insulin production that can be measured to see if a person's body is still producing insulin at all.

CSII—Continuous subcutaneous insulin infusion; a long term for pumping insulin.

Dawn phenomenon—An early-morning rise in blood glucose levels caused by a normal surge in growth hormones at this time of day.

Diabetes Control and Complications Trial (DCCT)—A nine-year study by the National Institutes of Health that showed that tight control improved the lives of people with diabetes.

Diabetic ketoacidosis—Severe high blood sugar in which the body searches out food from muscle and fat, thus over-spilling ketones. This condition requires emergency help.

Edmonton Protocol—A method of islet cell transplantation that uses more islet cells and a less-toxic combination of drugs to suppress the immune system. First used on adult patients with severe Type 1 diabetes at the University of Alberta, Edmonton, Canada, in June 2000, the protocol provides "proof of principle" that islet transplantation can potentially work.

Endocrinologist—A medical doctor who treats people who have problems with their endocrine system. The pancreas is an endocrine gland; diabetes is an endocrine disorder.

Glucagon—A hormone made by the pancreas that raises blood sugar levels. Available in shot form, it is injected during severe lows to avoid seizures.

Glucose—A simple sugar found in the body. Also known as dextrose, it is the body's main source of energy.

Glycosylated hemoglobin—The full name of A1c.

Honeymoon period—A period of time after diagnosis when the pancreas still produces some insulin. Can last weeks or years.

Humalog—Short-acting insulin used to cover meals and snacks; sometimes used in an insulin pump.

Hyperglycemia—A higher-than-normal level of glucose in the blood. Symptoms include frequent urination, excessive thirst, and weight loss.

Hypoglycemia—A lower-than-normal level of glucose in the blood. Symptoms include shakiness, weakness, pallor, hunger. It must be treated with carbs immediately.

Infusion set—The catheter, cannula, and insertion set used to connect an insulin pump to the body.

Insulin—A hormone secreted by the beta cells of the pancreas that helps the body convert glucose to energy in the cells.

Insulin pump—A small, computerized, and programmable device about the size of a beeper that can be used to deliver insulin to the body in place of injections.

Insulin resistance—Reduced insulin sensitivity by cells; usually the underlying cause of Type 2 diabetes.

Intermediate-acting insulin—An insulin such as NPH that peaks multiple times and stays in the body for at least twelve hours.

Islet cell—The cells in the pancreas that produce insulin. Pronounced "eye-let."

Islet cell transplantation—A still-experimental process of taking Islets from a cadaver and, via a portal injection, transferring them into the body of someone with diabetes.

Ketoacidosis—A serious condition in which the body does not have enough insulin and eats extra fat, spilling too many acidic ketones. Symptoms are thirst, frequent urination, and vomiting. This condition can cause coma and death.

Ketones—Acidic by-products of fat metabolism.

Lantus—A long-acting, nonpeaking insulin that stays in the body for as long as twenty-four hours, it is most often combined in use with a fast-acting insulin.

Logbook—A book or file used to track a child's blood sugar readings, food eaten, and activities.

Microalbuminuria test—A urine test that checks how the kidneys are working.

Neuropathy—Nerve damage caused by diabetes, usually at the extremities such as the feet and toes.

Novolog—A fast-acting insulin that can be used to cover meals and snacks, it stays in the body only about three hours.

Pancreas—The gland near the stomach that secretes insulin, glucagon, and digestive enzymes.

Pediatric Endocrinologist—An endocrinologist trained and licensed in the care of children with diabetes and other endocrine disorders.

Postprandial tests
A check of blood sugars about two hours after meals to see how the food made the blood sugar spike.

Reservoir—The plastic part of an insulin pump that holds the insulin.

Retinopathy—Renal eye disease, or damage to the nerves in the back of the eye caused by complications of diabetes and now very treatable with laser surgery.

Somogyi effect—A high blood sugar caused by a "bounce back" after an extreme low blood sugar.

Type 1 diabetes—Insulin-dependent diabetes in which the body's immune system has attacked the islet cells of the pancreas and the body makes little or no insulin. Replacement insulin is necessary for this type of diabetes.

Type 2 diabetes—A metabolic disorder in which the body still makes insulin but has trouble using it. It can be controlled by diet and exercise but does sometimes need insulin and other medications. Type 2 accounts for 95 percent of diabetes cases.

Appendix B

Top Diabetes Centers in Major Cities

Albuquerque

Presbyterian Hospital
201 Cedar SE, Suite 4640
Albuquerque, NM 87106
505-563-6530
www.phs.org

University of New Mexico Hospital
Department of Pediatrics
MSC10-5590
1 University of New Mexico
Albuquerque, NM 87106
505-272-5551
http://hospitals.unm.edu

Atlanta
Emory Children's Center
2015 Uppergate Drive NE
Atlanta, GA 30322
404-727-3708
www.emoryhealthcare.org

Pediatric Endocrine Associates
5455 Meridian Mark Road, Suite 520
Atlanta, GA 30342
404-255-0015
www.pedendo.tripod.com

Baltimore
Johns Hopkins Children's Center
600 North Wolfe Street
Baltimore, MD 21287
410-955-6463
www.hopkinschildrens.org

Sinai Pediatric Endocrinology
2411 West Belvedere Avenue
Baltimore, MD 21215
410-601-8331
www.lifebridgehealth.org

University of Maryland Medical Center
22 South Greene Street
Baltimore, MD 21201
800-492-5538
www.umm.edu

Boston

Children's Hospital Boston
Division of Endocrinology
300 Longwood Avenue
Boston, MA 02115
617-355-7476
www.childrenshospital.org

Joslin Diabetes Center
1 Joslin Place
Boston, MA 02215
617-732-2400
www.joslin.edu

Massachusetts General Hospital
55 Fruit Street
Boston, MA 02114
617-726-2000
www.mgh.harvard.edu

New England Diabetes & Endocrine Center
40 Second Avenue
Suite 170
Waltham, MA 02451
781-890-3610

UMass Memorial Medical Center
55 North Lake Avenue
Worcester, MA 01655
508-334-1000
✍*www.umassmemorial.org*

Chicago

Chicago Children's Diabetes Center
La Rabida Hospital
E. 65th at Lake Michigan
Chicago, IL 60649
800-770-2232
✍*www.larabida.org*

Children's Memorial Hospital
2300 Children's Plaza
Box 54
Chicago, IL 60614
773-880-4440

Northwestern Hospital
303 E. Ohio, Suite 460
Chicago, IL 60611
312-908-8023

University of Chicago
5758 S. Maryland Avenue
Chicago, IL 60637
773-702-6138

Yackgamon Children's Pavilion
Lutheran General Hospital
1675 Dempster Street
Park Ridge, IL 60068
847-318-9330

Detroit

Children's Hospital of Michigan (CHM)
3901 Beaubien
Detroit, MI 48201
313-745-KIDS (5437)
888-DMC-2500
✍*www.chmkids.org*

Helen DeVos Children's Hospital
100 Michigan Street NE
Grand Rapids, MI 49503
616-391-9000
✍*www.devoschildrens.org*

Houston

Memorial Hermann Children's Hospital
Pediatric Endocrine Clinic
6410 Fannin, Suite 500
Houston, TX 77030
832-325-6516
✍*www.memorialhermann.org*

Texas Children's Hospital
Diabetes Care Center
6621 Fannin Street, CC 1020.05
Houston, TX 77030-2399
832-822-3670
✍*www.texaschildrenshospital.org*

Los Angeles

Children's Hospital Los Angeles
4650 W. Sunset Blvd.
Los Angeles, CA 90027
323-669-4606
✍*www.childrenshospitalla.org*

Neufeld Medical Group Inc.
8733 Beverly Blvd.
Suite 202
Los Angeles, CA 90048
310-652-3976

White Memorial Pediatrics Medical Group
1701 Cesar E. Chavez Ave.
STE 456
Los Angeles, CA 90033
323-987-1200
www.whitememorial.com

Minneapolis
Children's Hospital and Clinics of Minnesota
McNeely Pediatric Diabetes Center and Endocrinology Clinic
345 N Smith Ave.
St Paul, MN 55102
651-220-6624
www.childrensmn.org

International Diabetes Center-Park Nicollet
3800 Park Nicollet Blvd.
St Louis Park, MN 55416
952-993-3393
www.parknicollet.com

Mayo Clinic
Division of Pediatric Endocrinology
200 First Street SW
Rochester, MN 55905
www.mayoclinic.org

Pediatric Specialty Clinic at University of Minnesota Children's Hospital
516 Delaware Street SE
Clinic 4A, 4th Floor
Phillips-Wangensteen

Minneapolis, MN 55455
612-626-6777
www.fairview.org

New York City
Mt. Sinai MC Pediatric Endocrinology
One Gustave Levy Place
8th Floor
New York, NY 10029
212-241-6936
www.mssn.edu

NYU Medical Center
530 First Avenue
New York, NY 10016
212-263-7300
www.med.nyu.edu

Schneider Children's Hospital
40 Lakeville Road
Suite 180
New Hyde Park, NY 11042
718-470-3290
www.schneiderchildrenshospital.org

Weill Medical College of Cornell University
525 E. 68th Street
Suite M-602
New York, NY 10021
212-746-3462
www.med.cornell.edu

Palm Beach
Broward Medical Center
Chris Evert Children's Center
1625 SE 3rd Ave., Suite 635
Ft. Lauderdale, FL 33316
954-764-0921
www.browardhealth.org

Joe DiMaggio Medical Center
Endocrine/Diabetes Center
1150 N. 35th Ave.
Hollywood, FL 33021
954-986-2234
✎ www.mhs.net

Pediatric Endocrine & Diabetes Specialists
3400 Burns Rd., Suite 100
Palm Beach Gardens, FL 33410
561-624-1985

Pediatric Endocrinology Consultants
5800 Colonial Dr., #205
Margate, FL 33063
954-968-8555

Phoenix

Phoenix Children's Hospital
1919 E. Thomas Rd.
Phoenix, AZ 85016
602-546-1000
✎ www.phoenixchildrens.com

Southwest Pediatric Endocrinology, PLC
10900 N. Scottsdale Road, Suite 504
Scottsdale, AZ 85254
480-991-2230
✎ www.swpedendo.medem.com

St. Louis
Saint Francis Hospital
I 55 & Route K
Cape Girardeau, MO 63701
573-331-5897

Saint John's Mercy Health Care
615 S. New Ballas Road
St. Louis, MO 63141
314-822-PEDS
✎ www.stjohnsmercy.org

Saint Louis Children's Hospital
One Children's Place
Suite 11E10
St. Louis, MO 63110
314-454-6051
✎ www.stlouischildrens.org

Southeast Missouri Hospital
1701 Lacey St.
Cape Girardeau, MO 63701
573-334-4822

University of Missouri Hospital, Columbia
Cosmopolitan International Diabetes Center
One Hospital Drive
Columbia, MO 65212
Administrative Office:
573-882-6979 or 800-500-6979

Tucson

University of Arizona
Angel Clinic
1501 N. Campbell Ave.
3rd Floor, # 3324
Tucson, AZ 85724
520-626-0381
✎ www.ahsc.arizona.edu

APPENDIX C

Sample Log Sheet

Monitoring Your Child's Blood Sugar Levels

A good log sheet, such as the example shown here, can make all the difference in tracking your child's care, trends, and needs. Log sheets can be used on paper, on a computer screen, even on a PDA. To find other samples and one that fits your need, check out these Web sites:

www.insulin-pumper.org
www.childrenwithdiabetes.com
www.dia-log.com
www.diabetesmanagementworks.ca

Or, ask your endo team for some samples. Parents who keep regular log sheets find diabetes care all the more reasonable.

Day	Blood Glucose Value	Carbs	Bolus	Correction	Notes
Monday					
7 A.M					
9 A.M.					
11 A.M.					
1 P.M.					
3 P.M.					
5 P.M.					
7 P.M.					
9 P.M.					

Tuesday

7 A.M.					
9 A.M.					
11 A.M.					
1 P.M.					
3 P.M.					
5 P.M.					
7 P.M.					
9 P.M.					

Wednesday

7 A.M.					
9 A.M.					
11 A.M.					
1 P.M.					
3 P.M.					
5 P.M.					
7 P.M.					
9 P.M.					

Thursday

7 A.M.					
9 A.M.					
11 A.M.					
1 P.M.					
3 P.M.					
5 P.M.					
7 P.M.					
9 P.M.					

Friday

7 A.M.					

9 A.M.					
11 A.M.					
1 P.M.					
3 P.M.					
5 P.M.					
7 P.M.					
9 P.M.					
Saturday					
7 A.M.					
9 A.M.					
11 A.M.					
1 P.M..					
3 P.M.					
5 P.M.					
7 P.M.					
9 P.M.					
Sunday					
7 A.M.					
9 A.M.					
11 A.M.					
1 P.M.					
3 P.M.					
5 P.M.					
7 P.M.					
9 P.M.					

Most parents check their child's levels eight times a day, but you should consult your medical team to help you decide how often is right for you.

Index

Alc (average blood sugar)
  about, 53–55
  good vs. bad, 59–61
  realistic goals, 58–59
  spikes in, 55
advocacy, 251–52, 254–62, 274
alcohol, 195, 233–34
American Diabetes Association
  (ADA), 253–55
amputations, 272–73
AntiCD-3, 271
appetite, 29
artificial pancreas, 267–69
attention issues, 105–7
attitude changes, 225–28
autoimmunity, 2–3, 6, 271
average blood sugar (Alc). *See* Alc
average lifespan, 61

babysitters, 115–16
Bag of Hope program, 167, 256
beach trips, 147–49
bedwetting, 4
behavior changes, 5
birthday parties, 145–47
blame, 218–19
blindness, 272
blood glucose checks
  bedtime, 57–58
  high readings, 99–101
  during honeymoon period, 180
  during illness, 244
  low readings, 101–2
  midday, 56–57
  morning, 55–56, 193
  nighttime, 57–58, 102–4, 193
  overdoing, 103
  playtime activities and, 135–36
  at school, 122–23
blood glucose meters, 69–71,
  73–77, 264–65, 268–69
blood glucose ranges
  Alc, 53–55
  daily averages, 55–58
  good vs. bad, 59–61
  initial, 36
  realistic goals, 58–59
  target, 54

bolusing, 86
bones, broken, 242–43
books, 173–74
breaks, 242–43
burnout
  age and, 210–12
  avoiding, 215–17
  battling, 204–7, 217–21
  in children, 201–12
  counseling for, 207–8, 221–23
  in parent/caregiver, 213–24, 262
  punishment vs. protection for, 207
  signs and symptoms, 201–4, 213–15
  support groups for, 209, 221
bus drivers, 131

camping trips, 150
camps, 168–70, 209, 217
carbohydrates, 9–10
caregiver burnout, 213–24, 262
caregiving roles, 112–15, 215–16
celiac disease, 38, 250
cell phones, 138, 150
Certified Diabetes Educators
  (CDEs), 40–41
chat rooms, 171–72
children
  burnout and, 201–12
  giving shots to, 30–31
  guilt and fear of, 33–34
  independence for, 189–200
  preteen, 58–59
  school age, 58–59, 165, 190–94, 211–12
  support for, 163–75
  therapy for, 174–75
  young, 58, 84–85, 164, 210–11.
  See also teenagers
Children with Diabetes, 156, 171, 257
cigarettes, 195
coaches, 141–42
colds, 239–40
cold weather, 138–40
college, 199–200
complications, 271–73
continuous glucose meters
  (CGMs), 73–77, 268–69
continuous subcutaneous insulin
  infusion (CSII). *See* insulin pumps

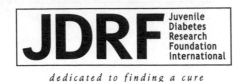

Take action!

The Juvenile Diabetes Research Foundation is an international group of parents just like you dedicated to a future free of diabetes and its complications. Getting involved is simple. Consider the following:

- **Get support!** Log onto *www.jdrf.org* and click on the On Line Diabetes Support Team to get help on issues, to have a Bag of Hope Delivered, or just to get some support.

- **Join the effort!** Log onto *www.jdrg.org* or call 1-800-JDF-CURE and get connected to your local JDRF chapter. There you can join the annual Walk to Cure Diabetes, attend support groups, help out with a Gala and more.

- **Become an advocate!** JDRF's Grass Roots Advocacy Program is considered one of the finest in Washington DC and across the nation. On May 17, 2006, JDRF's advocacy program was profiled on the front page of the New York Times. Among the many superlatives used to describe our program, the article said that "the foundation typically outperforms, in lobbying and fund-raising, nearly every other interest group built around a particular disease." It's easy to become an advocate. Just click onto www.jdrf.org/advocacy and follow the steps from there. As an advocate, you'll get regular updates about what's going on in Washington, and be asked to do anything from make a call or write a letter to an elected official, to actually meeting with them to tell your diabetes story.

Together, we will be known as the people who cured diabetes!